Camouflage

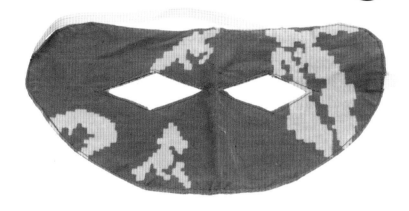

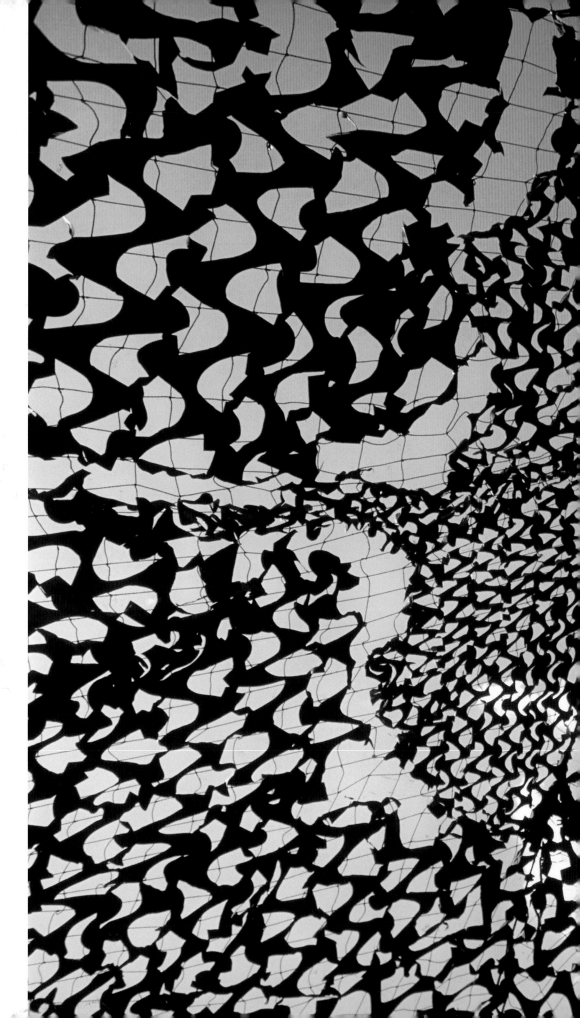

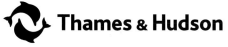
Thames & Hudson

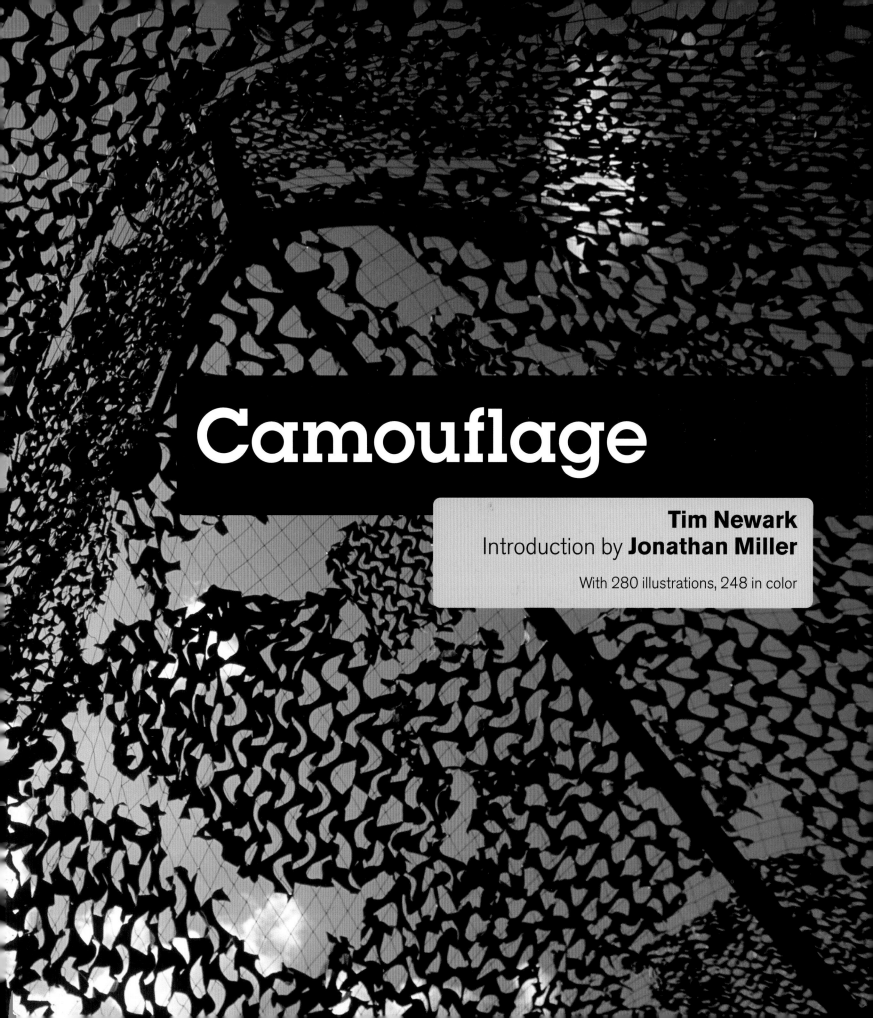

Camouflage

Tim Newark
Introduction by **Jonathan Miller**

With 280 illustrations, 248 in color

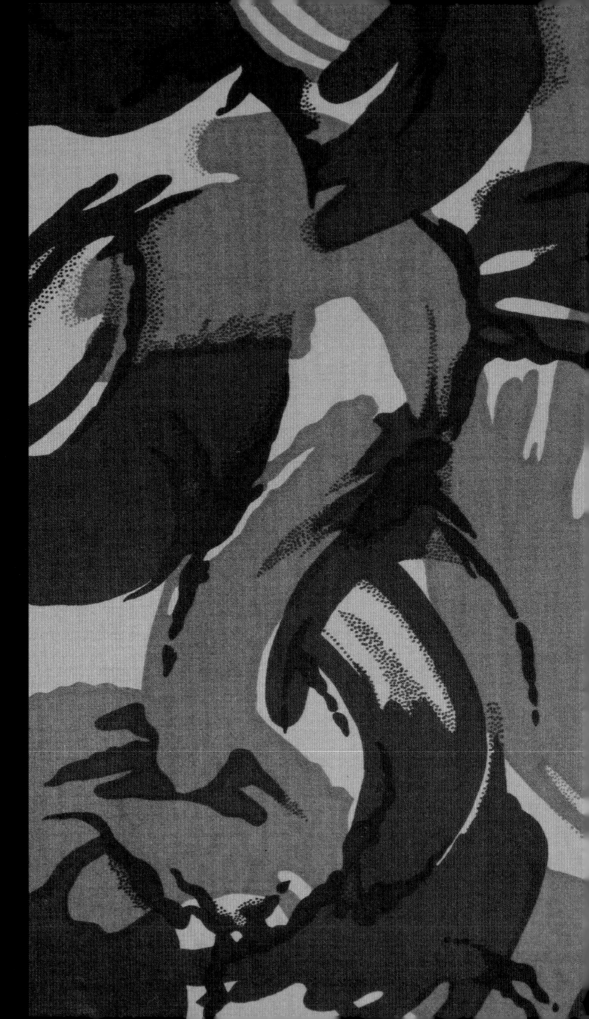

PAGE 1: Soviet sniper's face mask in a pattern known as KLMK, consisting of a light green background and random sand khaki 'pixel' shapes. Developed in the late 1960s, this pattern is believed to be a computer design.

PREVIOUS PAGES Camouflage netting on display during Desert Storm homecoming celebrations in Washington, DC, June 1991.

RIGHT British Army disruptive pattern material (DPM), the classic pattern of black, brown and green 'brush-strokes' on a light khaki background that was first issued in 1968.

OVERLEAF Venezuelan paratroopers participate in an Independence Day parade in Caracas, 6 July 2005.

Published in association with the Imperial War Museum, London. www.iwm.org.uk

First published in 2007 in hardcover in the United States of America by Thames & Hudson Inc., 500 Fifth Avenue, New York, New York 10110

thamesandhudsonusa.com

Library of Congress Catalog Card Number 2006908242

ISBN-13: 978-0-500-51347-7
ISBN-10: 0-500-51347-3

Printed and bound in China by Sing Cheong Printing Co. Ltd

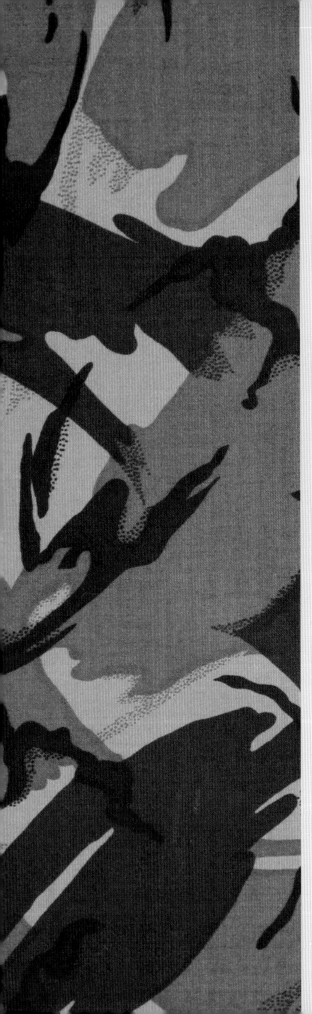

Contents

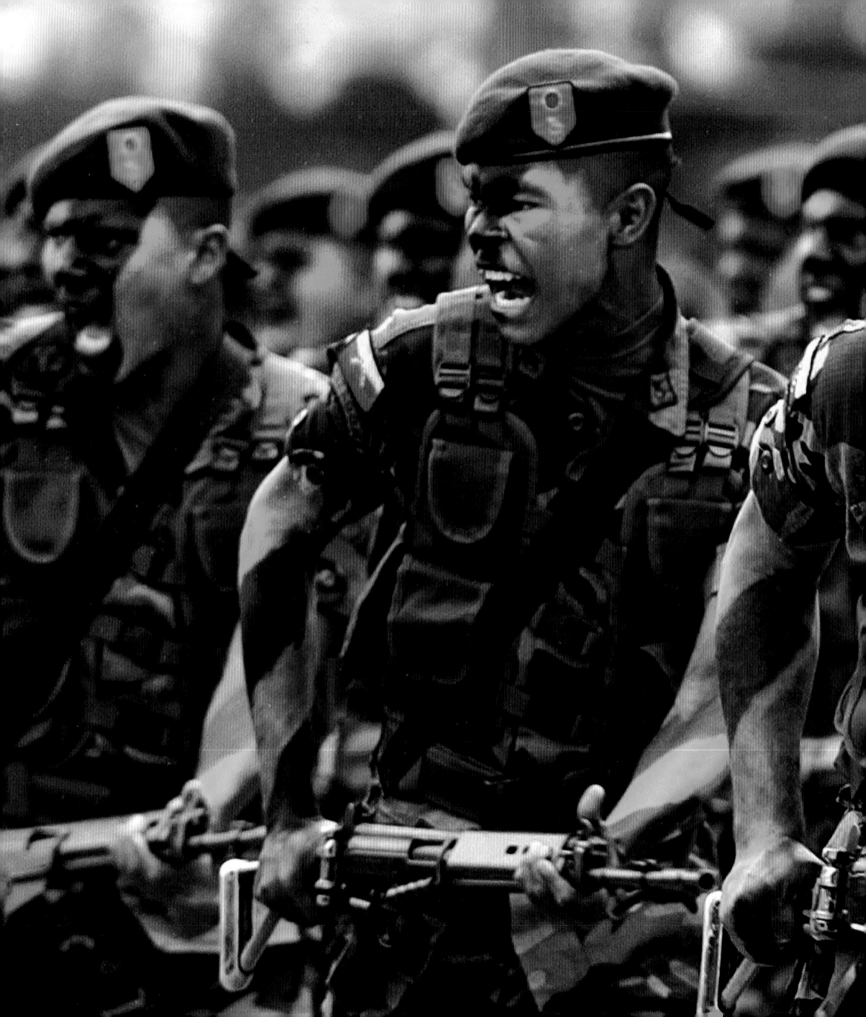

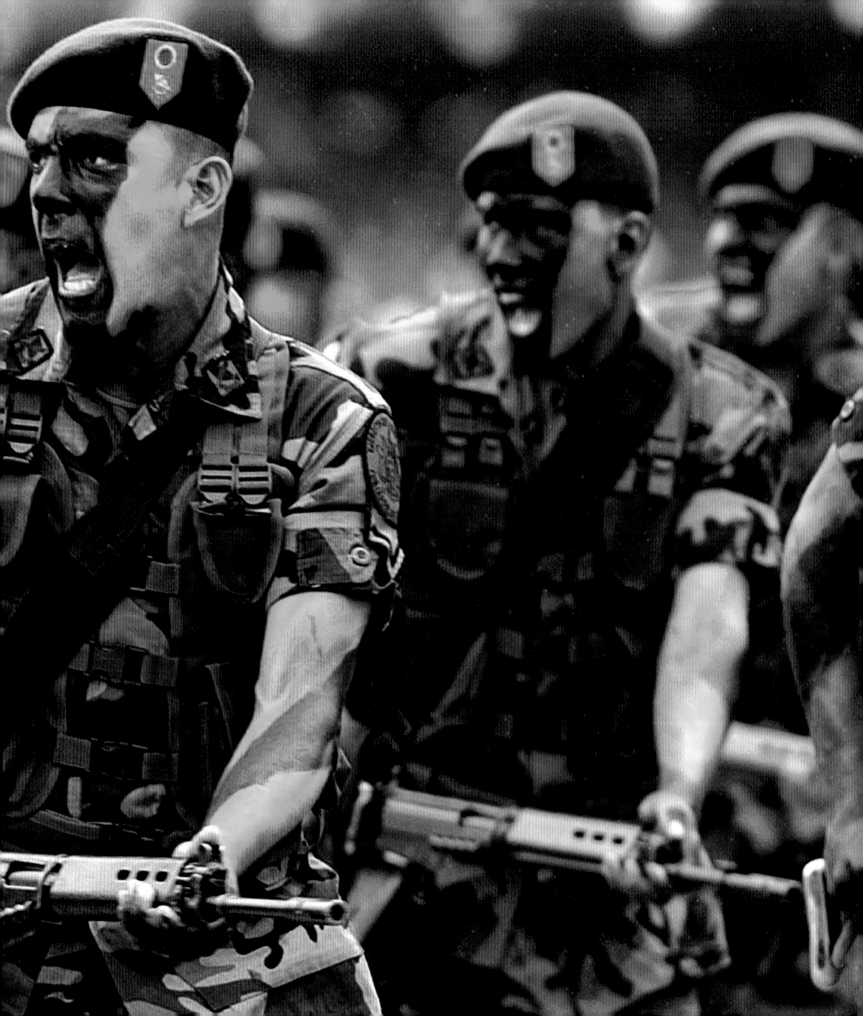

Preface

Camouflage has had an extraordinary impact on the art and design of the last hundred years. Born out of war in an age of machines, it takes its inspiration from nature. It is partly about being a chameleon – adopting the colours of a particular setting in order to blend in and become inconspicuous. But this is a limited strategy. Backgrounds are inevitably variable, and so movement is liable to give the game away. This is as true for a tank or warship as it is for a soldier or a tiger. One solution – in nature, as in war – is Disruptive Pattern. Areas of dark and light tone next to each other have the effect of breaking up shape and outline, especially when viewed from a distance. In the First World War, huge battleships were painted with disruptive pattern camouflage known as 'Dazzle' – outrageously bold, modernist designs that covered the ship's entire hull and superstructure and confounded all usual expectations of light, shade and form.

Camouflage is also about fooling the observer. In nature this might mean mimicking a stick, leaf or other unremarkable feature of the environment. In warfare it may mean the use of dummies and decoys such as the fleets of dummy tanks and aircraft that helped fool Hitler into believing that the Allied invasion of France in 1944 was to come at the Pas de Calais rather than Normandy.

By its very nature, camouflage has always attracted visual and creative talents, especially during the two World Wars. When Picasso saw camouflage-painted artillery in the streets of Paris in the First World War, he declared 'It is we who created that!'

In the second half of the 20th century the US intervention in Vietnam brought camouflage back into the popular consciousness. Above all this meant the disruptive pattern textiles that have not only become virtually synonymous with combat gear, but one of the most ubiquitous design motifs of our times.

By sporting camouflage gear, protesters against the Vietnam War were among the first to turn this symbol of militarism against the powers that created it. In the 1980s, US hip hop artists took up camouflage as an emblem of urban warfare and restless protest. In fashion, camouflage has appeared in both streetwear and couture. Numerous artists and designers have explored its potent and curiously contradictory associations.

For camouflage is both an emblem of military might and a symbol of subversion; a popular, even beautiful form of decoration that is also a tool of war; an abstract representation of the natural environment that was invented as a defence against deadly man-made machines. This book seeks to reveal its fascinating history.

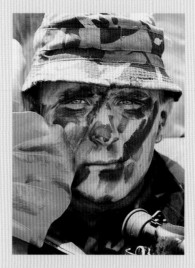

◄ **British infantryman** crouching in dense foliage wearing full camouflage including face cream. Exercise Red Stripe, Belize, June 1993.

▼ **Urban camouflage designs** by Adelle Lutz for the 1986 film *True Stories*, directed by David Byrne.

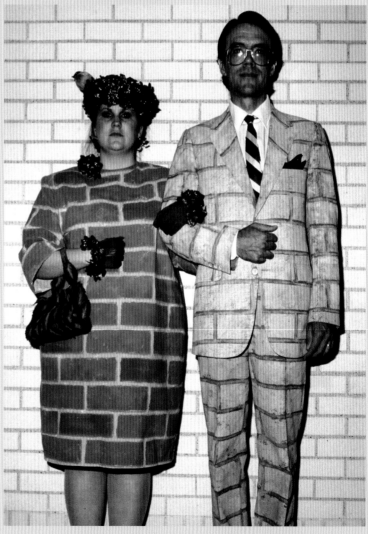

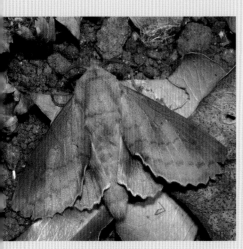

⬜ **A Lappet moth**, its rich red-brown colouring providing effective camouflage against a backdrop of earth and dead leaves.

▶ **Decorated camouflage jacket**, part of the Maharishi label's spring/summer 2004 recycled range. The 1960s London-based label Mr Freedom, famed for its psychedelic designs, was invited by Maharishi to apply its 'All You Need is Love' artwork to authentic Swedish and American military surplus garments. This US 'Woodland' pattern jacket bears lettering, hearts, stars, recyclable logos and a CND badge.

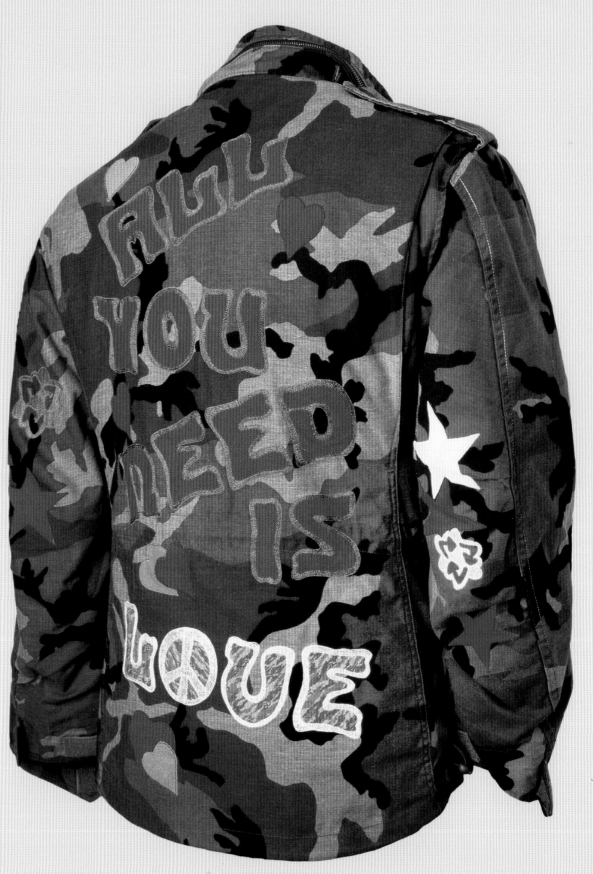

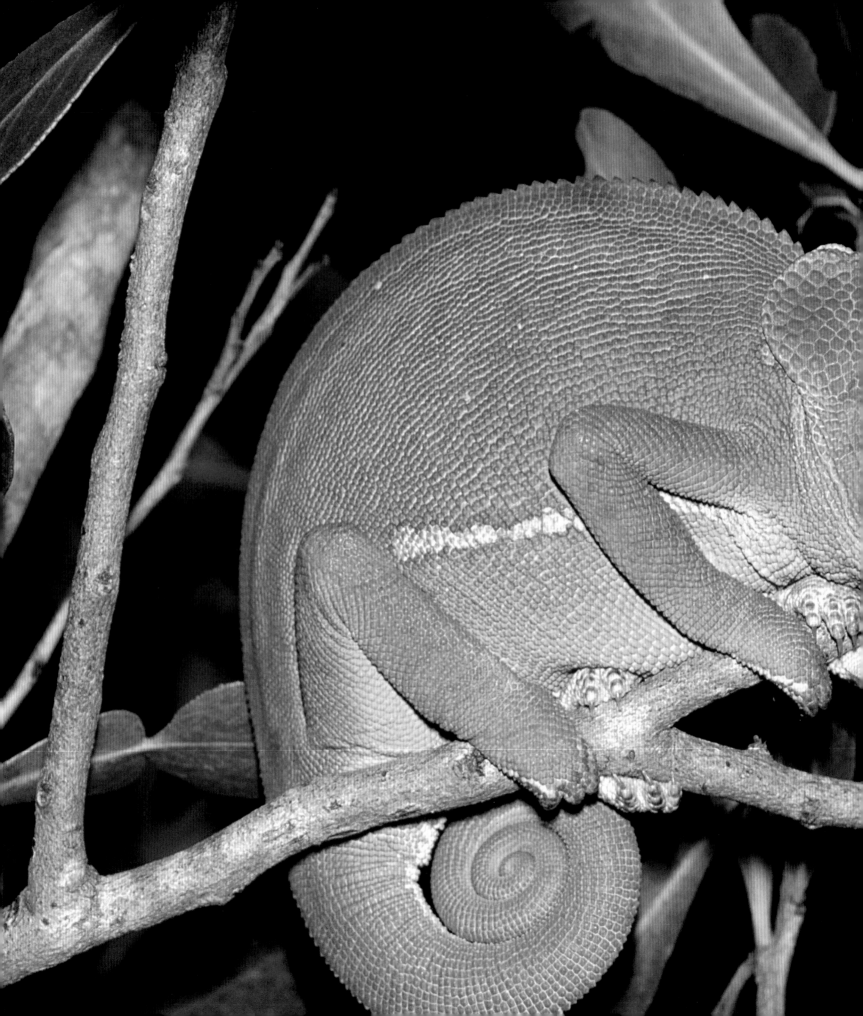

Visual Subterfuge in the Natural World

Introduction by Jonathan Miller

The animal kingdom is filled with creatures whose colours and patterns help conceal and protect them. By the time camouflage became a widespread military priority, the great naturalists of the 19th and early 20th centuries had already laid the groundwork with their pioneering studies of visual subterfuge in the natural world.

Visual Subterfuge in the Natural World
Introduction by Jonathan Miller

Previous page: Green chameleon in a tree. Certain fish, amphibia and reptiles possess the ability to change colour with remarkable speed and fluidity.

◪ **Shoal of sardines, New Zealand.** The 'silvering' of the body surface of some species of fish helps reduce their visibility to predators. The shiny scales reflect an image of the foreground, which at certain depths is more or less indistinguishable from the background.

Long before its military usefulness had been recognized and exploited under the now familiar but surprisingly recent title of 'camouflage', naturalists had repeatedly drawn attention to the biological use of visual subterfuge and to the fact that the form and colour of many animals serve the purpose of concealment and disguise. Throughout the 19th century the reports multiplied, but there was no comprehensive analysis of the subject until British zoologist Sir Edward Poulton published his fundamental work on *The Colours of Animals* in 1890, by which time – three decades after the publication of Darwin's *The Origin of Species* – it was almost unanimously accepted that these profitable adaptations were the unplanned results of natural processes, and not, as was once supposed, the products of purposeful design.

Like many of his predecessors, Poulton recognized that the colours and forms developed by living organisms could be either *protective* or *aggressive*, depending on whether they served 'to defend from attack or to assist in capture', and he went on to argue that in each case there were two relatively distinct ways of achieving the desired effect.

The first of these he described as a *general resemblance* to the variegated colours of the environment. Such a creature would, to some extent at least, blend in, as if it had become transparent, thereby affording an apparently uninterrupted view of the background. In fact, although Poulton doesn't refer to it in any detail, actual transparency is occasionally employed to achieve this cryptic effect. For optical reasons, it only works under water, but there are certain species of fish whose tissues have become so rarefied that their refractive index approximates to that of the surrounding medium, with the result that light passes through their bodies without noticeably betraying their slightly prismatic presence. But even then, true invisibility is compromised by the light-absorbing pigments of the eye and by the opacity of food in the gut.

'Silvering' of their bodily surface produces a comparable reduction in the visibility of certain fish, although in a completely different way. By reflecting, as opposed to transmitting, light, the shiny scales project an image of the foreground. At certain depths this image is relatively blurred and more or less indistinguishable from that of the background, with the result that the creature which furnishes this hazy reflection becomes conveniently inconspicuous.

Such effects involve modifications of the creature's body, but many animals achieve the same end by *constructing* whatever is required to hide themselves out of material salvaged from their environment. The caddis fly larva, for example, encrusts itself in a makeshift shroud of sand grains, small shells and vegetable bric à brac, as do certain sea urchins. Another example of such

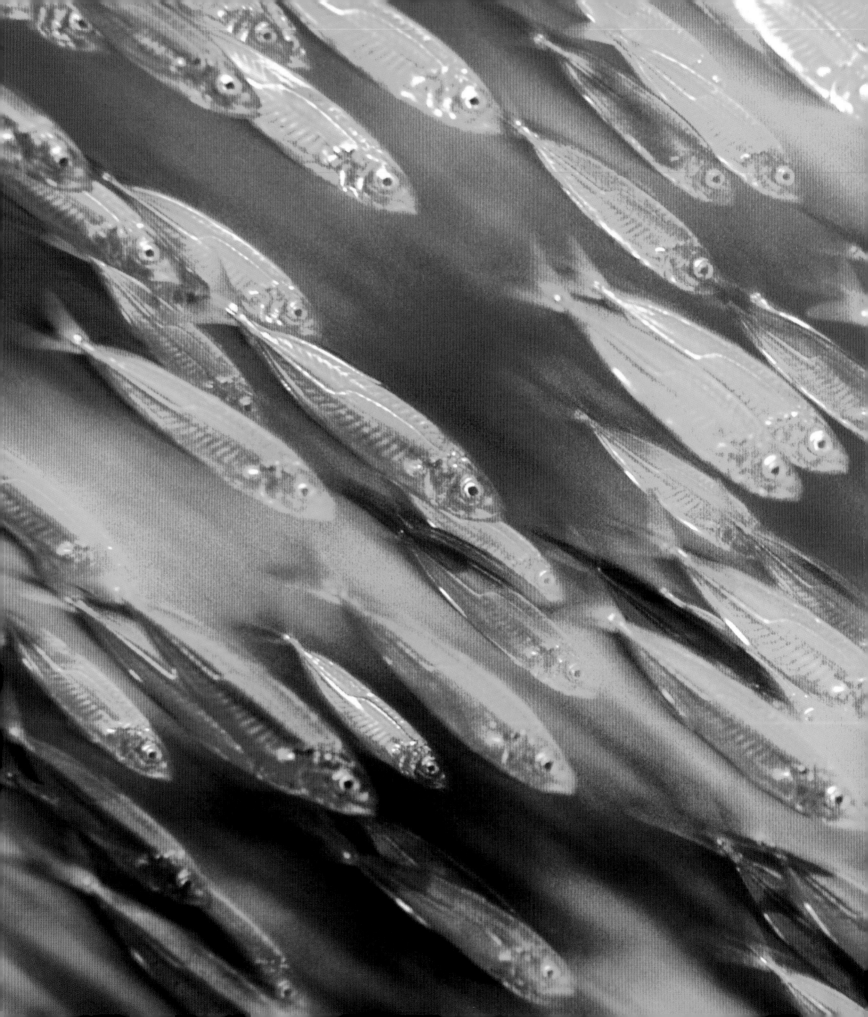

'adventitious' concealment was reported by the pioneering geneticist William Bateson. He described a species of crab which 'takes a piece of weed in his two [claws], and, neither snatching nor biting it, tears it across.... He then puts one end of it into his mouth, and, after chewing it up, presumably to soften it, takes it out and rubs it firmly on his head or legs until it is caught by the peculiar curved hairs which cover them.'

Purposeful though they seem, it would be a mistake to suppose that such disguises are assembled, in the way that military camouflage is, with the conscious intention of concealment. Because although there is an undeniable sense in which Bateson's crab *constructs* its artificial covering, just as the caddis worm does, there is neither intention nor ingenuity involved. In both cases, the actions which create the artefact are impulses dictated by genetic instructions inherited from the creature's ancestors – the same type of instructions that determine the creature's equally distinctive morphology. Like the spider's web or the bird's nest, they are examples of what Richard Dawkins calls the 'Extended Phenotype'. That is to say, they are the extended expression of the creature's inherited genotype.

In contrast to these kinds of disappearing tricks, there are certain creatures, especially insects, which remain perfectly visible, but disguised as something else. They assume what Poulton termed a *special resemblance* to a particular item on the scene. That is, they appear as something other than themselves – a dead leaf, say, a lichen-covered twig or even a bird dropping. Ideally, such disguises render a defenceless creature uninteresting to a hungry predator, and when employed by a predator give it a better chance of ambushing its prey undetected. For example, whereas ordinary caterpillars possess five pairs of legs, the so-called 'stick caterpillar' has only two at the rear end, with which it attaches itself to a twig, while its long thin body, which is corrugated with humps and bumps resembling irregularities of the bark, sticks out an acute angle from the stem, thus resembling an inedible branch. The stick caterpillar practises *protective* mimicry; as an example of *aggressive* mimicry, Poulton cites a Javanese spider which takes advantage of the fact that butterflies in that region are attracted by bird dung. According to the reports of a local naturalist, the spider resembles this alluring material in extraordinary detail. As soon as the unsuspecting prey alights on what it supposes to be its meal, it is trapped and devoured.

The success of such disguises depends on the ability of a creature to maintain a convincingly lifeless stillness, since any sign of liveliness would automatically give the game away. Nevertheless, given that it is not in fact a stick or bird-dropping, the creature must occasionally risk mobility in order to forage and mate. Hence stick

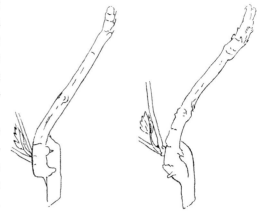

Larva of the swallow-tail moth, as illustrated in Sir Edward Poulton's *The Colours of Animals*, the first comprehensive analysis of animal patterning and coloration, published in 1890.

Great spiny stick insect (below) and green stick insect (right). Like the swallow-tail moth larva, these insects practice what Poulton termed *protective* mimicry: they assume a resemblance to a specific feature of their environment that is of no interest to potential predators.

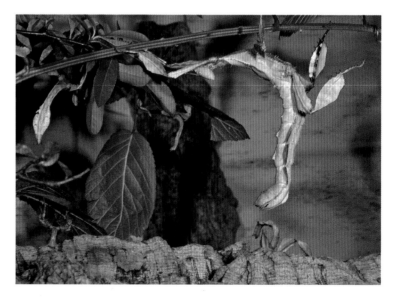

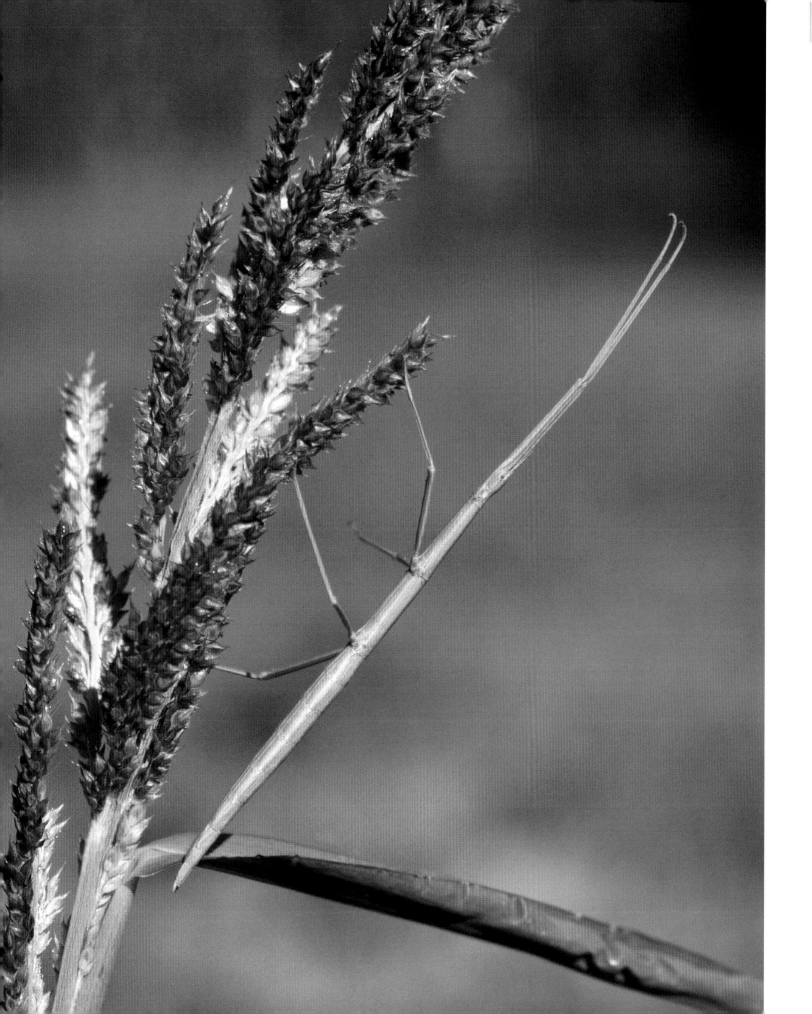

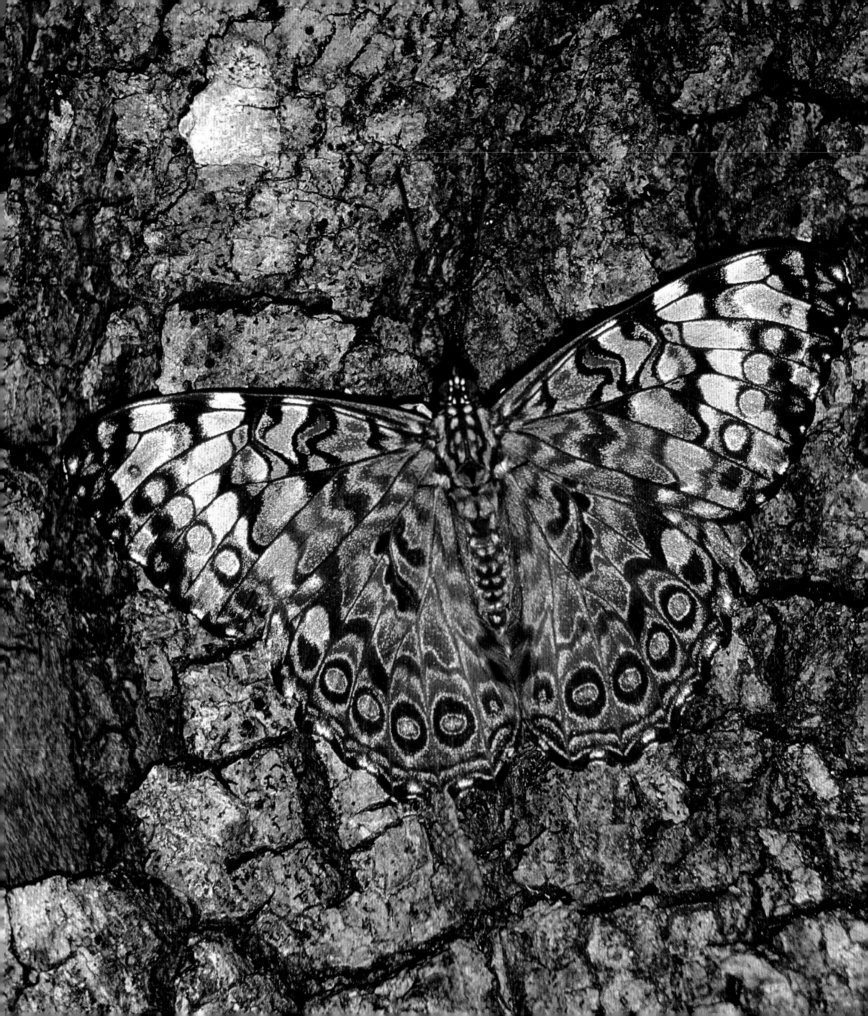

caterpillars pass themselves off as motionless twigs during the day and only relax their statuesque pose and crawl about to feed unseen under cover of darkness.

Compared to the often remarkable deceptions which can be achieved by mimicking the appearance of particular items in the environment, the alternative strategy of pretending not to be there at all is fraught with difficulties. Because even if the creature is sluggishly confined to one particular habitat, wearing patterned colours which blend into those of its immediate surroundings, a careless movement will immediately betray its presence. Species which assume a general resemblance to their chosen environment therefore frequently reinforce their concealment by developing the ability to stay motionless for long periods.

Creatures can achieve much more effective concealment by actually changing their appearance according to their setting. Poulton identified two ways in which this is achieved. *Discontinuous variations* are periodic transformations, often involving radical redesigns of bodily structure, which afford a creature the opportunity to blend in with a different setting. Such a strategy is more or less confined to butterflies and moths, whose characteristic metamorphoses from larva, through chrysalis to winged adult may coincide with abrupt changes in habitat. These episodic adjustments sometimes involve switching from a *special*

◁ **Bark-mimic butterfly resting on bark.** Creatures bearing patterns that merge with those of their habitat frequently reinforce the protection this affords them by developing the ability to stay perfectly motionless. Careless movement is dangerously eye-catching and a tell-tale sign of life.

▽ **Crab spider on a flower head.** This creature practises *aggressive* as opposed to *protective* mimicry. Crab spiders have the ability to change colour over a few days to match that of a particular flower head; or they will select a flower to match their existing colour. Either way, the spider waits there, motionless and inconspicuous, ready to ambush any insect that alights.

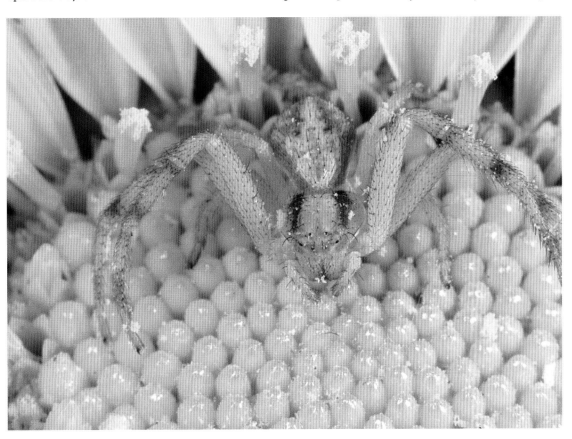

resemblance, in which the larval grub mimics the appearance of a twig or a rolled-up dead leaf, to a subsequent *general resemblance*, in which the winged adult assumes the overall colours of its background.

Certain fish, amphibia and reptiles possess the ability to change colour with remarkable speed and fluidity. Poulton categorized such rapid changes of appearance as *continuous variations*. Although the detailed mechanism by which these transformations are achieved was not fully understood at the time, Poulton and his contemporaries recognized that they were not, as might easily have been suspected, the direct result of variously coloured light 'imprinting' itself reversibly on photosensitive pigments in the skin. Experiments had proven that blinded animals lost the power of altering their colour to correspond with the surrounding hues, indicating that the effect was mediated indirectly through the eye, from which, according to Poulton, 'differing nerve impulses pass along the optic nerve to the brain. The brain being thus indirectly stimulated originates different impulses, which pass from it along the nerves distributed to the skin, and cause varying states of concentration of the pigment in the cells.'

In Poulton's day, as he admitted, 'the highest powers of the microscope have failed to detect the connection between the nerves and the pigment cells in the skin.' These connections can now be clearly viewed, yet the precise means by which a pattern projected onto the retina brings about a corresponding alteration of colours in the skin still remains a mystery.

The ability to realize such rapid changes of appearance, however they may happen, is confined to species whose versatile skin is sufficiently exposed to display them. The fur and feathers with which mammals and birds are clothed rule out the possibility of such conveniently prompt responses. Nevertheless, seasonal climatic changes are almost invariably accompanied by alterations in the colour of pelts and plumage. These often occur before there is any visible change in the appearance of the landscape, making it seem reasonable to assume that they are brought about not by visual stimuli but by a change in temperature. Once these seasonal coats have been established they remain unalterable until the time comes for them to undergo their replacement. The result is that the colours which succeed one another from one season to the next are inevitably generalized, and although they undeniably afford a significant degree of concealment – why else would they have been selected? – the extent to which they resemble each of the particular backgrounds in which the creature happens to find itself is inevitably limited. So again there remains a tendency to exploit stillness or stealth, sometimes both. Certain predators for example await motionless until their victim

▶ **Illustrations by the American painter and naturalist Abbott Thayer** showing a 'mirror-back caterpillar', 'crumple-leaf caterpillar' and 'curled dead-leaf caterpillar', all examples of what Sir Edward Poulton classified as *protective* mimicry.

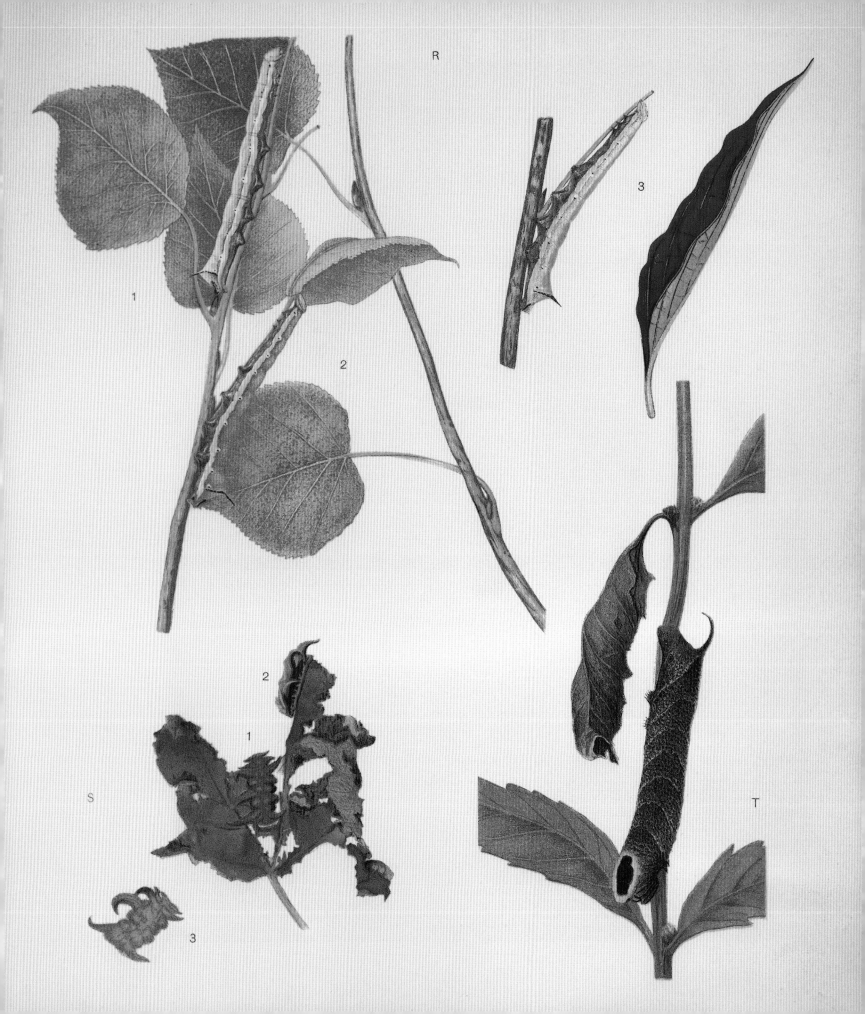

R

1

2

3

S

2

1

3

T

3

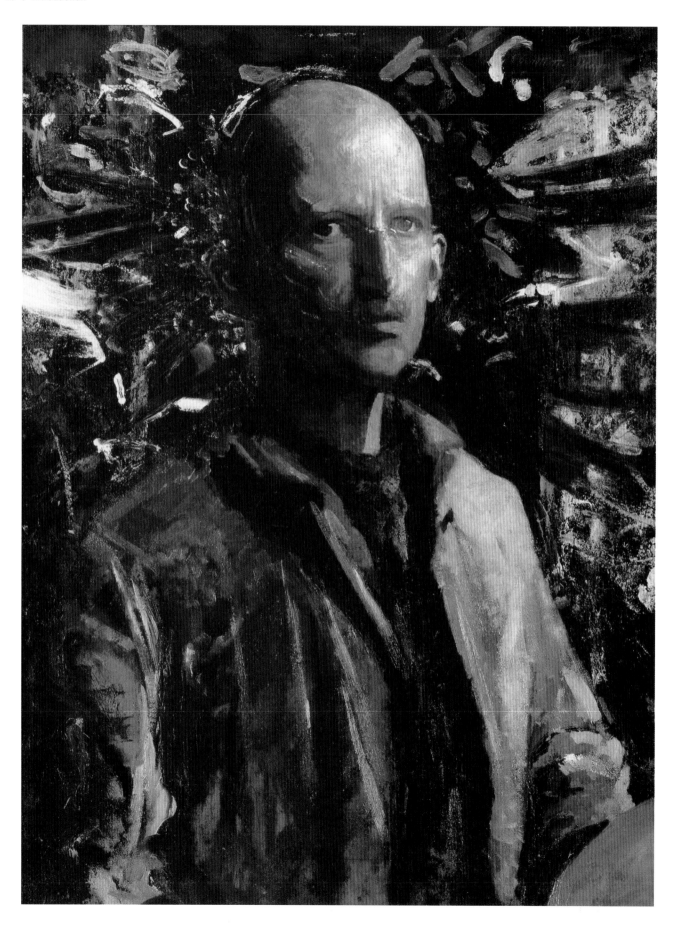

comes within reach of an easy snatch. Others actively stalk their prey, occasionally freezing if they have reason to suspect that their stealthy approach has been detected.

But there is another problem, and it applies, or so it is claimed, to any creature whose bulk is sufficient to expose it to the potentially revealing effects of being illuminated from the sky above. With its top side brightly lit and its underside in shadow, its three-dimensional presence, motionless or otherwise, becomes perilously apparent, regardless of correspondence, however close, to the colours and patterns of the environment.

Poulton believed that nature had developed an effective way of minimizing this particular risk of detection. By exploiting mutations which darken the illuminated top side while bleaching the dimly lit underside, he argued that natural selection had created a strategy to diminish the otherwise noticeable bulk of the creature. Although Poulton is rightly credited with the first account of this supposedly concealing device of 'counter-shading', the subject was broached at about the same time by the American naturalist and painter Abbott Thayer, who represented its usefulness with almost obsessional enthusiasm. According to him, artists knew better than anyone that differential shading was the most effective way of rendering the three-dimensional bulk of an object, so that it was only to be expected that nature would protect creatures by favouring variations which worked in the opposite direction. As far as he was concerned, counter-shading brought about a flattening effect which reduced a creature's otherwise bulky visibility. The fact that it was conspicuously absent in animals that lived in the dark confirmed his belief.

And yet the extent to which this principle achieves the flattening, let alone the concealing, effect which Thayer claimed is somewhat questionable. In many cases the transition from dark to pale takes place so far down on the creature's flank that the pallor in which it terminates is almost invisible. The result is that when the creature is viewed from the side, the counter-shading, such as it is, is all but hidden and so can make no significant contribution to its concealment.

Even when the gradation of tone is more clearly apparent, its flattening effect is debatable. Its advantage is certainly clear in the case of fish, which because they live suspended in water may be viewed by potential predators from above or below. When viewed from above, a fish's dark top side will blend into the dimness of the unilluminated depths; conversely, a white underside seen from below will blend into the brightness of the sky above. The same principle applies to the colouring of certain birds. But in fact neither of these are true examples of counter-shading, for the simple reason that a dark back or light underside is only effective in helping to conceal the creature when the other is not

◄ *Self-Portrait* **by Abbott Thayer, 1920.** Thayer believed passionately that his artist's eye and training enabled him to interpret with authority the coloration and shading of animals.

▼ **A bobcat perched in a tree.** Many animals have a lighter underside that graduates into darker shades on their sides and back. Thayer believed that this 'counter-shading' was a protective device to diminish the three-dimensional bulk of a creature when viewed from above or at distance.

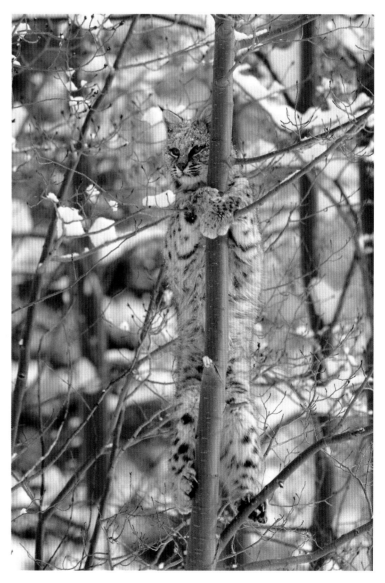

visible. They make independent contributions to concealment; the fact that there happens to be a graded transition between them is all but irrelevant.

In spite of these and other objections, the concept of counter-shading continued to play a prominent part in the various theories of cryptic coloration and its importance was repeatedly stressed by the naturalists who succeeded Poulton and Thayer, especially by the distinguished British zoologist Hugh Cott in his classic 1940 study, *Adaptive Coloration in Animals*. Cott also emphatically stressed its practical importance in his subsequent work on military camouflage during the Second World War (see pages 101–2).

During the years that Thayer continued to publish his over-stated claims with regard to counter-shading, his attention was drawn to a less questionable type of natural concealment – one which would shortly play a significant part in the subsequent development of military camouflage. He observed that the variegated colours which afford many creatures a generalized resemblance to their surroundings are often supplemented by patches, stripes and blotches whose abrupt shapes break up the contours by which they would otherwise be identified. Given the fact that the concealment achieved by resembling the background is unavoidably partial, these 'disruptive' patterns provide

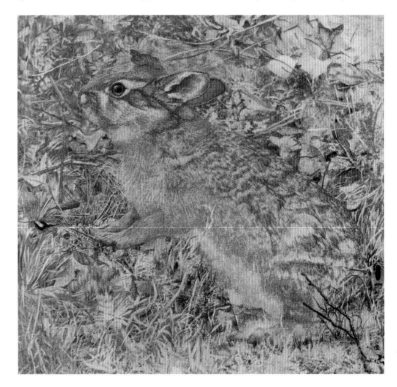

▶ **Illustration of a rabbit by Abbott Thayer**, from his book *Concealing Coloration in the Animal Kingdom*, 1909. The variegated colours on its back allow it to blend in with its grassy habitat, while the graduated shading towards a lighter underbelly represents 'counter-shading'. Thayer was a close observer of the natural world, but he also at times used his considerable artistic skills to reinforce his arguments about the working of colour and pattern in the animal kingdom.

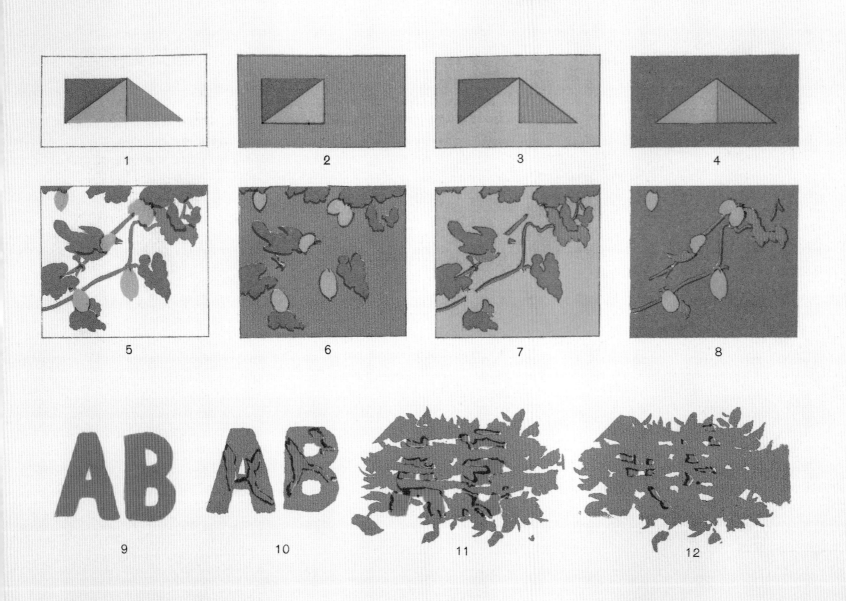

▲ Diagram by Abbott Thayer demonstrating the principle of 'disruptive coloration'. Thayer observed that patches, stripes and blocks of colour in an animal's markings have the effect of visually breaking up its contours, making it more difficult to distinguish at a distance.

a helpful note of confusion, if only because they serve to divide the attention of the observer between a number of conflicting shapes among which it is less easy to distinguish that of the creature itself.

Thayer's recognition of 'disruptive coloration' anticipated its theoretical formulation by the Gestalt psychologists of the early 1920s. These German investigators were preoccupied with the principles which determine the recognizability of natural objects and abstract shapes. According to them, one of the factors which make a 'figure' distinguishable from the 'ground' against which it is seen is its coherent unity and the fact that its contours enclose an unambiguous 'form' or 'Gestalt'. Anything which competes with the legible continuity of its outlines would compromise its salient identity.

It's easy to see how suggestive these ideas would have been to anyone who was interested in the ways in which animals conceal themselves, though as it happens, Thayer died just before the fundamental works in Gestalt psychology were published and discussed. But even if they had been published earlier it is unlikely that he would have acquainted himself, let alone sympathized with, these somewhat abstract arguments. For as far as he was concerned the truth of the matter was self-evident to anyone who worked in the visual arts. In the introduction to the 1908 edition of

◹ **A male ruffled grouse** in its forest habitat. Illustration by Abbott Thayer from his book *Concealing Coloration in the Animal Kingdom*, 1909.

◸ **A hog-nosed viper**, whose disruptive pattern allows it to merge with the dead foliage that litters the ground of its rainforest habitat.

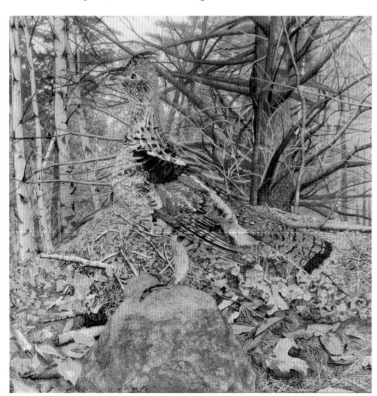

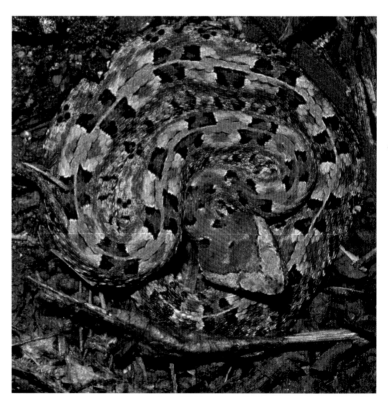

▼ **A Siberian tiger** hidden amongst tall grasses and twigs.

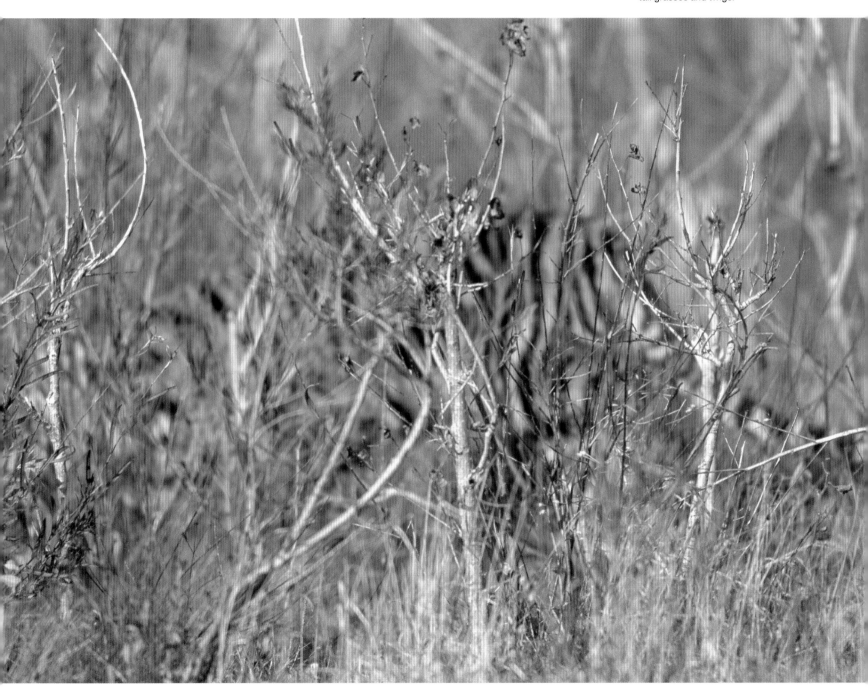

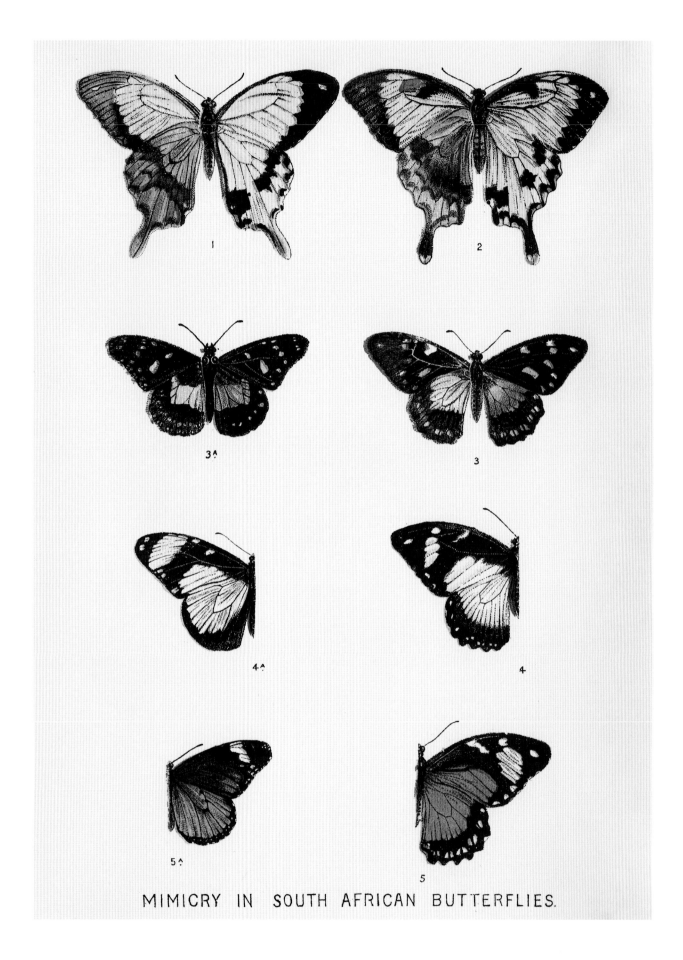

MIMICRY IN SOUTH AFRICAN BUTTERFLIES.

his *Concealing Coloration in the Animal Kingdom* he announced that the subject had got into 'the hands of the wrong custodians' and that 'it properly belongs to the role of pictorial art, and can be interpreted only by painters. For it deals wholly in optical illusion and this is the very gist of a painter's life.'

As a result of this proprietorial attitude, Thayer failed to take any account of the by then widely reported fact that 'disruptive colours' sometimes made creatures more rather than less conspicuous, and that this was not necessarily to their disadvantage. For example, in 1867 Alfred Russel Wallace had already explained to Darwin's satisfaction that colourful ostentation was sometimes a beneficial feature. If a species happened to combine conspicuous coloration with prickles, poisons or a repulsive taste, predators would eventually learn the costs of attacking it. By bearing the tolerable loss of a few individuals, the species as a whole, and the bold colours that singled its members out, would eventually gain a protectively deterrent reputation.

A few years later Wallace's colleague H.W. Bates drew attention to an interesting variation on this theme. He reported the existence of edible species whose conspicuous appearance mimicked that of unpalatable ones. Without having to incur the biochemical expense of developing poisons, their striking resemblance to species which had done so would, in the course of time, lend them the vicarious reputation of being too costly to attack. However, the efficiency of this device presupposes that the palatable species are outnumbered by their unpalatable counterparts.

In 1879 the German naturalist Fritz Müller drew attention to an alternative version of the mimicry which Bates had recently described. He identified a number of equally unpalatable insect species, all of which displayed the same conspicuous uniforms, thereby spreading the risks of educating hungry predators.

Although Poulton took some time to accept the statistical evidence in favour of Müllerian mimicry he immediately recognized the importance of Wallace's findings, not to mention those of Bates. Unlike Thayer, he acknowledged the fact that concealment was not the only way of reducing the risk of being attacked, and that as long as there was memorable correlation between the appearance of a creature and its unpleasant taste, the very fact that it was conspicuous would play a significant part in the defence of its fellows.

In contrast to the various forms of concealment and mimicry mentioned earlier – for which, as we shall see, there are many recognizable counterparts in human warfare – it is difficult to identify any military equivalents to the 'warning colours' described by Wallace, Bates and Müller. Although a conspicuous show of armed strength does often play a significant part in disconcerting the enemy, the threat which is represented by such displays is

◁ **Mimicry in South African butterflies**, an illustration from Hugh Cott's *Adaptive Coloration in Animals*. The butterflies labelled 3, 4 and 5 are perfectly edible, but protect themselves by their resemblance to inedible species 3a, 4a and 5a. This particular type of mimicry was first identified by the naturalist H.W. Bates.

intended to create alarm, whereas in the case of 'warning' colours there is nothing intrinsically deterrent about their appearance. On the contrary, they positively invite the greedy attentions of a predator, whose subsequent reluctance to attack such self-advertising prey depends on the ability to remember the unpleasant consequences of doing so. And even then, the tutorial effect is confined to the individual predator unlucky enough to suffer such a bitter experience.

Meanwhile Wallace had already identified yet another benefit to be gained by undertaking the risks of being conspicuous. But in this case the value lay in attracting the attention of individuals of the same species as opposed to that of its enemies. 'Gregarious mammals,' for example, 'while they keep together, are generally safe from attack, but a solitary straggler becomes an easy prey to the enemy; it is therefore of the highest importance that the wanderer should have every facility for discovering its companions with certainty at any distance within the range of vision.' In other words, the vividly noticeable colours shared by members of a particular species make it easy for them to recognize one another, so that if a particular individual strays into vulnerable isolation, it can readily identify the distant presence of its fellows and return to the collective security of the herd.

In this particular case there is, surely, a military equivalent to what Wallace describes. In traditional warfare at least, the existence of vividly recognizable uniforms and flags undeniably helped to maintain the disciplined coherence of the action. But since they also provided the enemy with a conveniently visible target, it's not surprising that with the introduction of smokeless powder and more accurately aimed firearms, conspicuous uniforms were soon replaced by drably inconspicuous khaki.

There was another example of conspicuous coloration which taxed naturalists during the 19th century. The frequency with which the males and females of a species differ in their appearance had many times been noted. In birds and insects especially, the females are reticently coloured, whereas their male counterparts display flamboyantly ornamental liveries. For Darwin, such differences were inconsistent with his theory of natural selection, because although there was an obviously protective advantage in the modest dress of females, it was difficult to understand why the male of the species exposed himself so flagrantly. As evolutionary historian Helena Cronin points out, 'Darwin came to the conclusion that natural selection was powerless to account for such apparently pointless splendour. His solution was his theory of sexual selection. He held that male ornamentation evolved simply because females preferred to mate with the best-ornamented males. This obviously gives these males a mating advantage and ultimately the likelihood of greater reproductive success. Thus,

▶ **Frontispiece from Hugh Cott's** *Adaptive Coloration in Animals.* Published in 1940, this classic work remains one of the most definitive studies of the subject. During the Second World War, the zoologist Cott brought his expertise to bear on military matters, when he worked for the British Army as an adviser and instructor on camouflage (see pages 101–2).

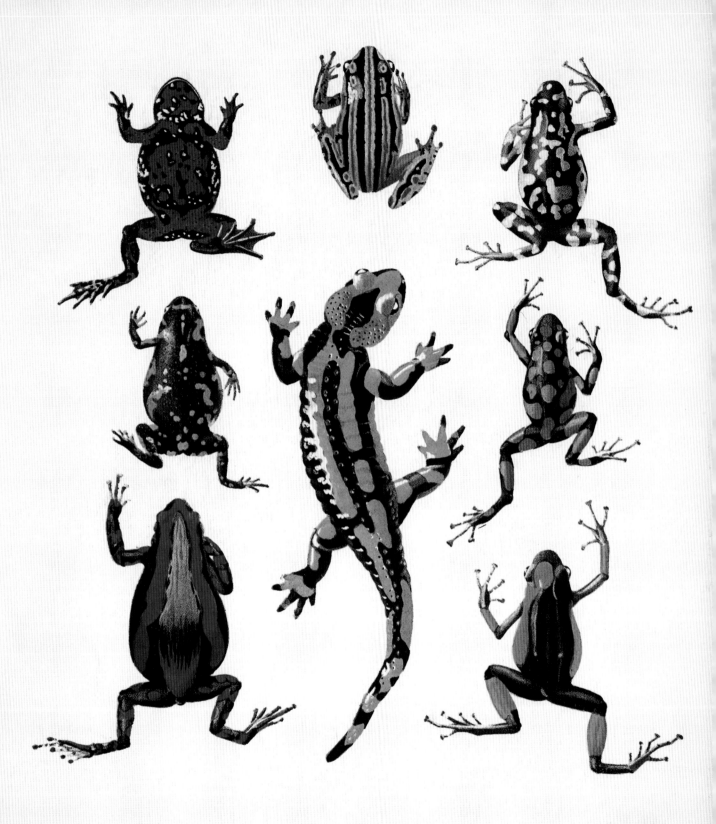

Hugh B. Cott *pinx*.

Bombinator igneus

Atelopus stelzneri

Phrynomerus bifasciatus

Hyperolius marmoratus

Salamandra maculosa

Dendrobates tinctorius

Dendrobates tinctorius

Dendrobates tinctorius

over evolutionary time, males develop ever-more exaggerated, immoderate flamboyance.'

To begin with, Wallace went along with this idea, but since it conflicted with what he regarded as the more fundamental truths of *natural* selection, he became increasingly reluctant to recognize the equivalent reality of *sexual* selection, and as time went on his disagreement with Darwin became more and more explicit. As far as he was concerned, bright colours were the natural expressions of health and vitality – witness the vivid tints of blood, bile and fat – and it was only when, in the case of brooding females, they were vulnerably exposed to the necessities of concealment that natural selection suppressed them in favour of more reticent appearances.

Wallace was by no means alone in this respect. In the years which followed its publication in the *Descent of Man* (1871), Darwin's theory of sexual selection was subject to widespread criticism and ridicule. Meantime the role of *natural* selection itself was also increasingly called into question, especially after 1900, when the rediscovery of Gregor Mendel's plant breeding work inaugurated the explosive growth of experimental genetics. For the practitioners of this new science, *mutation* – that is to say, abrupt and often large-scale change in the hereditary mechanism – was regarded as the driving force of evolutionary change, and the effect of selection was confined to the elimination of harmful novelties.

It took more than thirty years, but eventually there was a reaction against this attitude, epitomized by the polemical introduction contributed by Julian Huxley for Hugh Cott's *Adaptive Coloration in Animals*, published in 1940: 'Among a certain section of experimental biologists...it has been fashionable and indeed almost a matter of professional conscience to display a radical scepticism on the subject of adaptations, especially colour adaptations and most particularly mimetic adaptations. Upholders of the theories of protective and warning coloration and of mimicry have often been attacked as 'armchair theorists', insufficiently acquainted with modern work in genetics, which for some unexplained reason is held to do away with adaptive interpretations.' According to Huxley, 'Dr Cott, in this important book has turned the tables with a vengeance on objectors of this type... far from genetics in any way throwing doubts on their adaptive interpretation, the facts of cryptic, warning and mimetic coloration pose searching questions to the geneticist, and demand a recasting of many current views on the efficacy and mechanisms of selection.'

Cott's book is, as Huxley writes, a worthy successor to Edward Poulton's earlier work. It retains and adds to the categories established by his predecessor, and since natural history had flourished in the intervening years, undeterred by the condescension of laboratory scientists, Cott's text contains a wealth of previously unrecorded detail, copiously illustrated with many of his own accomplished drawings and photographs. In contrast to Poulton, his analysis is characterized by repeated reference to the optical principles involved in concealment and disguise:

'When we recognize anything by sight...the means by which the eye is enabled to distinguish it are fourfold, and it is essential for the proper understanding of our subject that these should be clearly appreciated. Firstly, the object appears in the field of vision as a continuous area of colour, differing more or less markedly in hue and purity and depth from its immediate surroundings, against which it is therefore seen to stand out in contrast.

Secondly, the (object) is not seen simply as a wash of flat colour – even when in actual fact it may be uniform in colour. For it is thrown into relief by the effect of light and shade, which enables the eye to detect surface curvature, modelling and texture.

Thirdly although natural objects are not, or are but rarely bounded by lines – in the way that an outline drawing is – nevertheless the surface of every visible body is framed by a contour [which] has a characteristic...shape, enabling the form of a familiar object to be recognized.

Fourthly, under certain conditions of illumination a shadow will be thrown by the object upon its background.... By framing the outline of the object, as well as by virtue of their own shape and conspicuousness, shadows tend to facilitate recognition.'

It is interesting to see how Cott applies some of these principles to what he regarded as the most important type of natural concealment, 'Disruptive Coloration' – a concept which had already influenced the development of military camouflage:

'Provided an animal is seen against a broken background, it is probably true to say any pattern of darker or lighter colours and tones will tend to hinder recognition by destroying to a greater or less degree its apparent form...but in order to achieve effective results the colours, tonal contrasts and patterns employed must conform to definite optical principles.... In the first place the effect of a disruptive pattern is greatly strengthened when some of its components closely match the background, while others differ strongly from it. Under these conditions, by the contrast of some tones and the blending of others, certain portions of the object fade out completely while others stand out emphatically'. As a result of this interaction between strongly contrasted adjacent tones, some of which blend into the background, the creature's recognizable identity is effectively disintegrated, so that instead of seeing one recognizable animal the observer is confronted by a clustered array of discontinuous surfaces. The effect is enhanced by disruption of the contours of the creature by means of patches

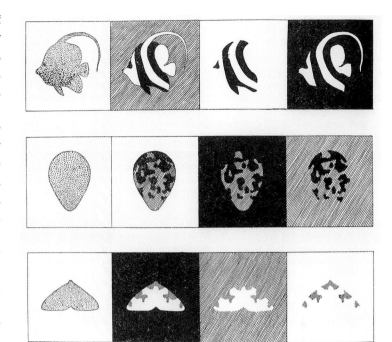

▲ ▼ **Illustrations from Hugh Cott's *Adaptive Coloration in Animals*,** 1940, demonstrating the principles of differential blending (above) and disruptive contrast (below). Cott analysed in authoritative detail the optical principles involved in concealment and disguise. He particularly emphasized the importance of 'Disruptive Coloration', in which patterns of darker and lighter colours have the effect of visually breaking up a creature's outline, making it harder for a predator to sight from a distance.

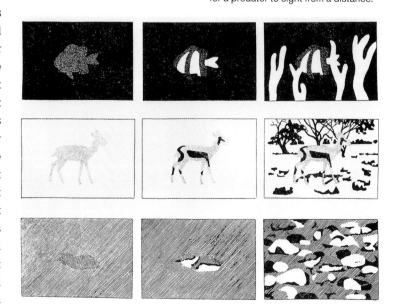

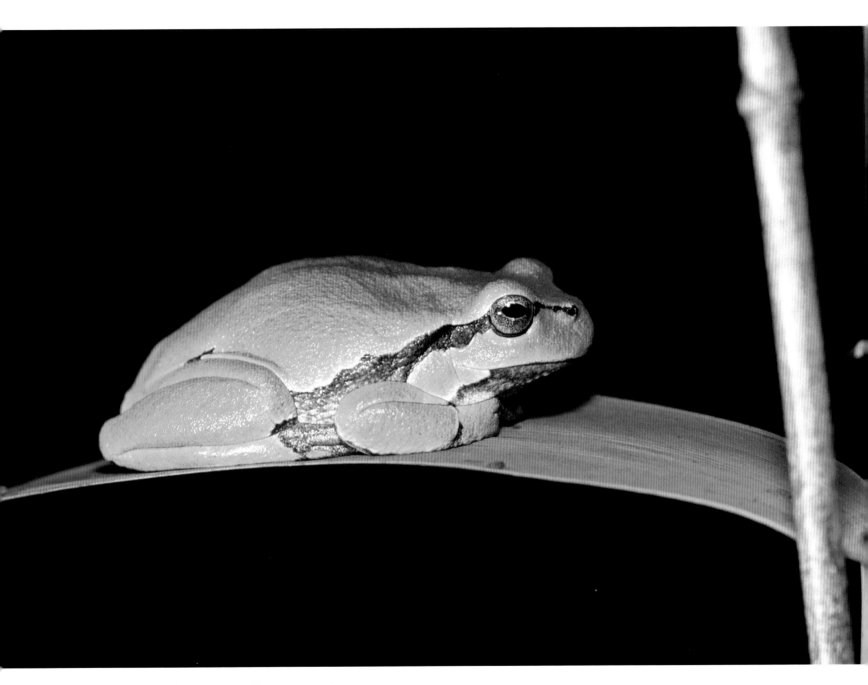

◪ A European green treefrog.
Hugh Cott observed that the markings on many frogs appear random when their legs are splayed, but align to form disruptive patterns when folded in to their bodies.

◪ During fieldwork in Portuguese West Africa Cott noticed that the patterns on certain species of frog formed coherent stripes when their legs were folded in, making the creature's outline much harder for any potential predator to distinguish. He called this phenomenon 'Co-incident Disruption'.

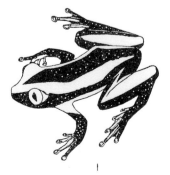

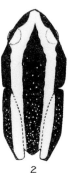

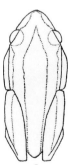

1

2

3

or stripes which cut across as opposed to running parallel to its all too recognizable edges.

In 1935 Cott read a paper to the British Association for the Advancement of Science in which he reported an important but previously unnoticed variation on this theme. He referred to it as *Co-incident Disruption*. During fieldwork in Portuguese West Africa, he had noticed that certain species of frog could increase the confusion created by their disruptive colours by bringing their striped limbs into close contact with comparably coloured stripes on the side of their body. With its thigh hugged close to the flank, 'the silvery stripe on the exposed part of the hind limb exactly coincides with, and forms an extension of, the similar stripe on each side of the back.' In this attitude, against a dark background, all that can seen is a dim blob with two parallel white stripes. Something similar happens when the common frog bends and folds up its hind legs: blotches and stripes which seem to have no relationship with one another when the limbs are extended line up to create a bewilderingly disruptive pattern.

The same principle is frequently exploited to reduce the conspicuousness of a vertebrate's eyes. As Cott observed, 'Of all shapes a round disc is the most striking and easily seen and recognized – hence the use of the "bull's-eye" for target practice.' Small though it is, the vertebrate eye with its dense black pupil stands out from the most jumbled background and thereby draws attention to its owner's vulnerable front end, where it can least afford the risk of injury. It's not surprising that nature has evolved a variety of 'disruptive' solutions to this problem. 'Animals belonging to many widely different families and orders have the eyes camouflaged in precise detail.... Sometimes an irregular dark disruptive area includes the whole orbit. Sometimes the upper margin of an elongated patch of dark pigment crosses the iris exactly on the top of the pupil...or again, the eye may be crossed by a stripe exactly the width of the pupil itself,' and so on.

Since the creature's front end is the one at which a predator's attack is most likely to prove fatal, Cott demonstrated that nature often provides a conspicuous *false* eye at the rear end, where injury would be somewhat less devastating. Poulton had, in fact, already identified such deflecting eye-spots in many species of butterfly. Other naturalists had demonstrated the frequency with which areas of the wing bearing such false eye markings show signs of damage from predators' attacking beaks.

And so it goes on for almost five hundred pages of such carefully analysed detail that it seems uncharitable to question Huxley's claim that it represents the last word on the subject. Nevertheless, to the modern reader it seems slightly odd that Cott expressed so little interest in how these adaptations might have come about during the course of the creature's development.

☑ **The eye of a vertebrate, with its dense black pupil,** stands out from the most jumbled backgrounds, as Cott's illustration demonstrates. This increases a creature's vulnerability to attack at its front end – precisely where damage is most likely to prove fatal.

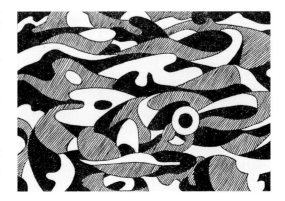

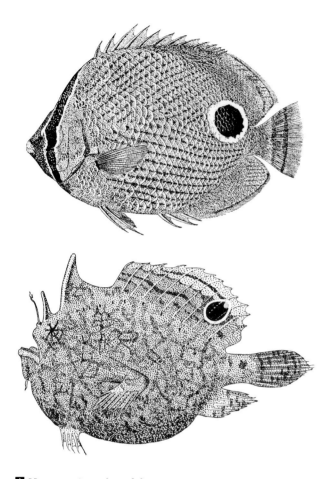

◿ **Many creatures bear false eye spots** on parts of their bodies where attack is less likely to prove fatal than if a predator were to target the real head and eye.

To some extent of course such considerations would have been irrelevant to the task he had set himself. As a dedicated naturalist he was concerned to analyse the usefulness of the various features he described; the question of their embryological origin was a distraction that in any case remained at that date unanswerable.

Biologists in the 1930s were already acquainted with the reproductive significance of chromosomes, and with the fact that the information which dictated the structure and function of the forthcoming organism was distributed throughout the length of these divisible filaments in the form of discrete, albeit invisible entities called genes. However, the medium in which this productive information was represented and the process by which it was translated into developmental effects remained obscure. In the last twenty years the relationship between molecular biology and experimental embryology has become so complex that it is impossible to provide a reasonable summary here. But research in this area has been so productive and so precise that scientists can now ask what were previously unanswerable and indeed inconceivable questions about the origins of the adaptations that Cott described sixty years ago.

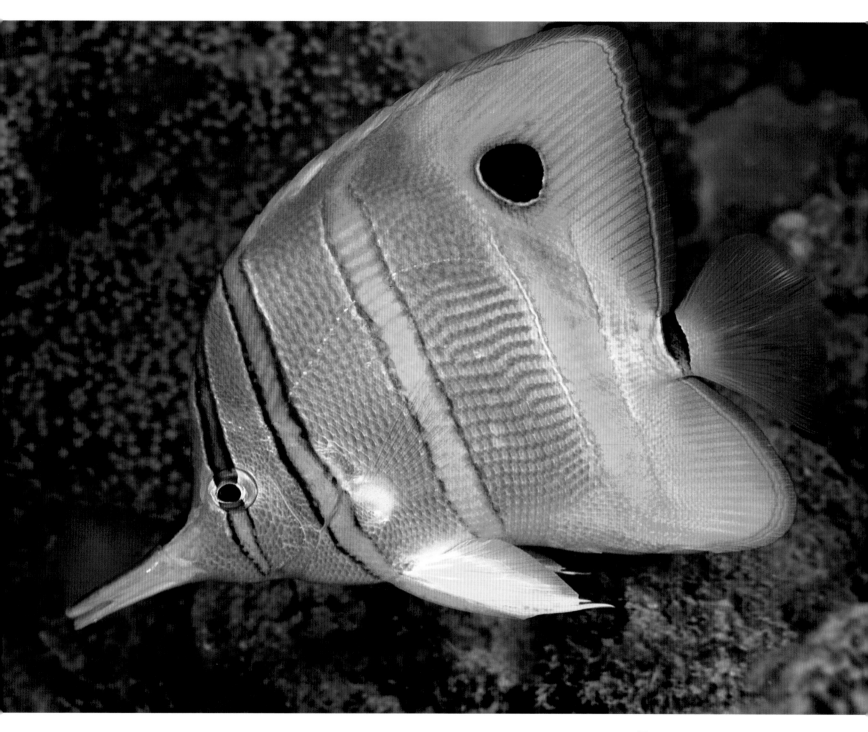

◩ **The beaked butterfly fish** has a prominent false eye spot at its rear end and a disguising band of colour that runs through its real eye.

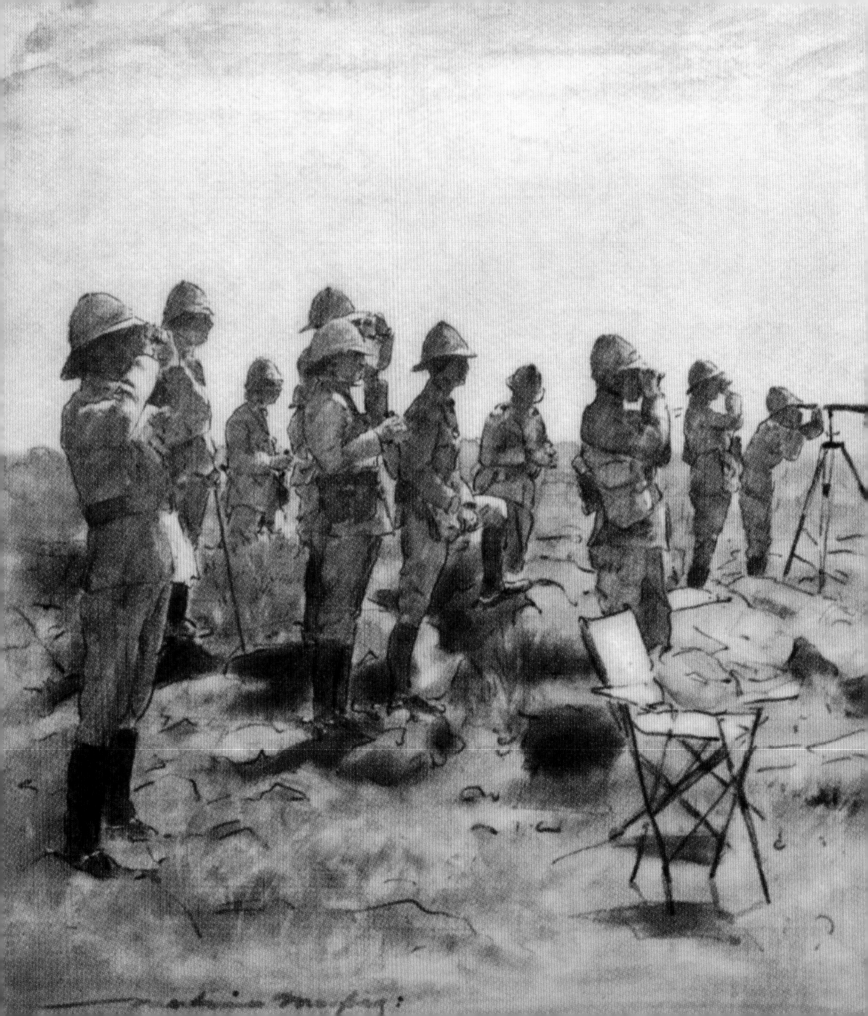

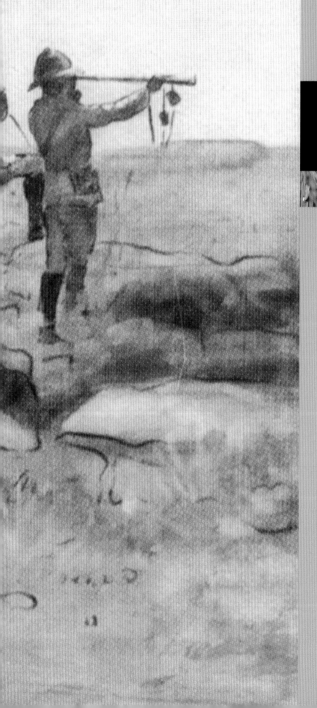

Hunters and Riflemen
Early Camouflage

Skilled hunters make skilled warriors, so it is no coincidence that the earliest military camouflage grew from hunting traditions. Even so, the greys and greens worn by 18th- and 19th-century sharpshooters remained largely the preserve of elite soldiers until colonial rebellion and the First World War made all too clear the need for uniforms that allowed modern soldiers to blend in, not stand out.

Hunters and Riflemen
Early Camouflage

Previous page: Khaki uniforms
were adopted for use on all British
overseas service in 1896. Here, Lord
Roberts, commander-in-chief of the
British Army, and his staff observe
a battle during the Boer War of
1899–1902. From Mortimer Menpes'
War Impressions, published 1901.

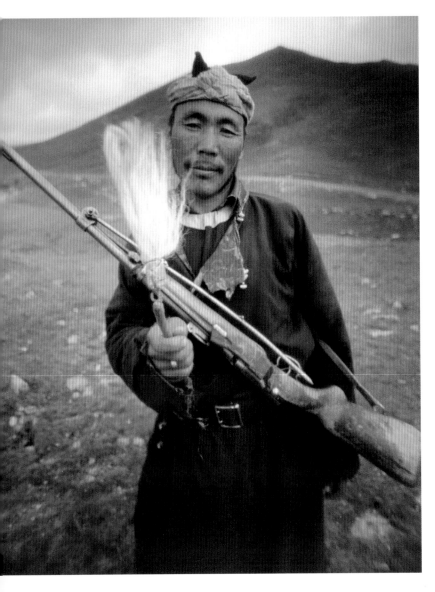

◄ **A Mongolian marmot hunter,**
wearing a hat with ears and carrying a
yak tail to entice his prey, demonstrates
the affinity of hunters with the natural
world around them.

The earliest wearer of camouflage was the hunter. In order to get close to his prey, prehistoric man needed to disguise himself. He would smear himself in mud to reduce his own scent and dull his shiny skin. He would clad himself in the local foliage. Sometimes he would wear the skin and fur of his intended prey or decorate his scalp with feathers.

Two kinds of hunting evolved, and with them two kinds of hunting attire that reflected the principal forms of camouflage in the animal kingdom. A hunter-stalker with a bow or sling might conceal himself completely in the landscape, waiting for hours to pounce. In this form of hunting he might disguise his presence with an outfit made of hundreds of strips of cloth that resembled the foliage around him. Certainly he would be likely to choose green or brown dyed clothing. Other hunters would operate in groups, working together to approach and spear an animal. In this they might choose not to resemble their background, as that would be constantly changing, but to break up their individual silhouettes. Thus they might paint their bodies with contrasting stripes in an intuitively grasped form of disruptive pattern camouflage similar to the natural markings on many of the predators they hunted.

The transforming of a hunter's appearance had a spiritual as well as practical dimension. Some primitive hunters believed they could acquire the speed, stealth or prowess of the animals they hunted if they wore their skins and copied their actions. Such rituals are believed to be depicted in rock paintings around the world.

The skills learned to track and hunt animals became the same skills needed by warriors to surprise their human enemies. Hunters therefore made skilled fighters and the tradition of hunter-soldiers has continued throughout history.

In his introduction to *Fieldcraft, Sniping and Intelligence*, published in 1940, Colonel Lord Cottesloe declared: 'What indeed is the human animal in war but a special variety of soft-skinned dangerous game?'

'The hunter of big game at home or abroad,' he said, 'has learnt by experience not only to make certain of the shot he fires, but to approach his objective unseen, to observe tracks and signs and all else within his ken.... Such a man has acquired in a high degree the qualifications of a very efficient individual soldier.'

It was the hunter-soldier who would be the very first professional warrior to wear camouflage.

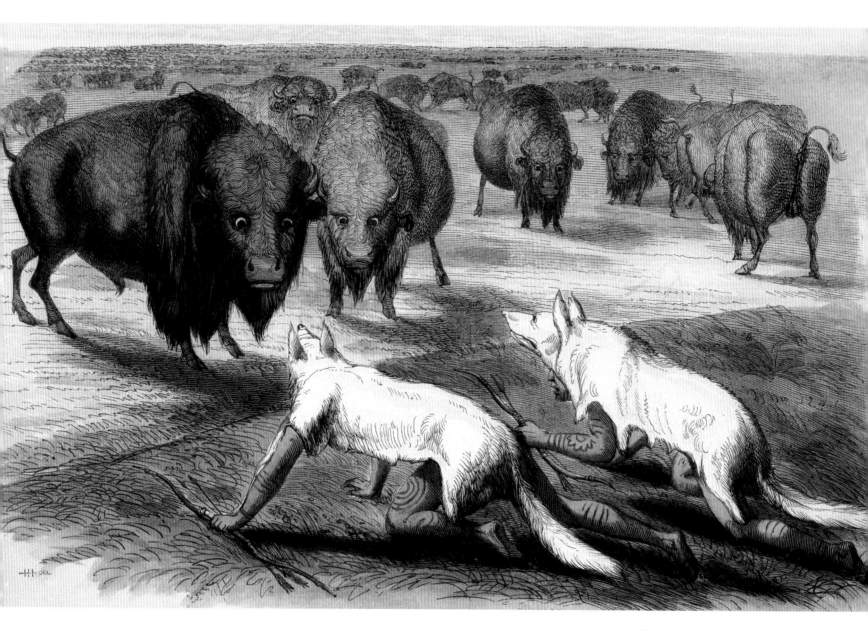

◤ **Native American hunters** wear wolf skins to stalk buffalo. The first wearers of camouflage were hunters. Sometimes they clad themselves in the skins of predators, believing they would acquire the strength and skills of those animals. Woodcut after George Catlin, 1840.

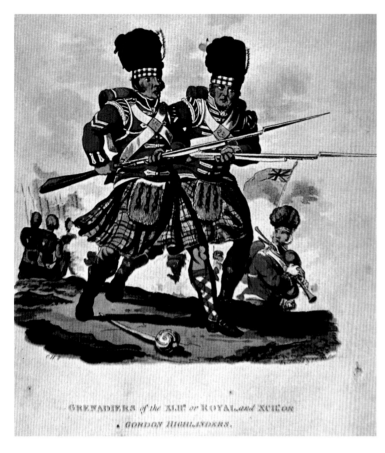

GRENADIERS *of the* XLII.^d *or* ROYAL *and* XCII^d *or*
GORDON HIGHLANDERS.

◢ **Black Watch and Gordon Highlanders** of 1812 drawn by Charles Hamilton-Smith. They combine British Army scarlet jackets with their traditional tartan kilts.

▶ **Government Tartan**, the dark green and black pattern worn by the Black Watch, the oldest of the British Army's Highland regiments.

Green Soldiers

Is tartan a form of camouflage? The popular red Royal Stewart sett seems an unlikely aid to concealment, but the properties of its intricate weaves and patterns make its earliest forms very sympathetic to the landscape it emerged from. Tartan today has come to be a largely Scottish phenomenon, but in prehistory it was worn by a wide variety of people, most likely Caucasian and of Celtic origin. The discovery of tartan textiles on preserved bodies in central Asia demonstrates that these Celtic peoples travelled far, and ancient Roman writers made reference to their chequered clothing.

In Britain, in the highlands of Scotland, one of the earliest recorded forms of tartan was a black and green striped pattern widely worn by Celtic clansmen. This eventually became the basis for what was known as the Government Pattern, worn by Highland warriors in the British Army. This dark pattern was perfectly matched to the volcanic rock mountains of Scotland with their sparse tufts of hardy greenery. It was worn in the form of a combined kilt and cloak, consisting of one long piece of fabric secured around the waist and then slung over the shoulder. Not only did it protect the wearer from the weather, but it also served as a blanket for sleeping under.

An explicit reference to tartan being worn as camouflage was recorded by Scots humanist George Buchanan in his *Rerum Scoticarum Historia* of 1582. He noted that Scots 'delight in variegated garments, especially stripes, and their favourite colours are purple and blue. Their ancestors wore plaids of many colours, and numbers still retain this custom, but the majority now in their dress prefer a dark brown, imitating nearly the leaves of the heather, that when lying upon the heath in the day, they may not be discovered by the appearance of their clothes.'

William Shakespeare dramatized one of the earliest uses of camouflage in warfare in his play *Macbeth*. He describes medieval Scottish warriors ripping down the branches of trees to disguise themselves as they march on an enemy castle: 'Let every soldier hew him down a bough/ And bear 't before him; thereby shall we shadow/ The numbers of our host and make discovery/ Err in report of us.'

Such a use of camouflage was rare in ancient and medieval warfare because, generally speaking, warriors did not need to disguise themselves. They fought hand to hand with spears and swords, and unless they were preparing an ambush, most warriors could not avoid being seen by their enemies. This type of open warfare continued even after the advent of firearms. For although the use of gunpowder weapons created a distance between lines of soldiers, the range of these early guns was not long enough to enable soldiers to hide and fire at the same time. This changed with the invention of the rifle.

▼ **The most famous literary reference to early camouflage** is William Shakespeare's description of Scots warriors using foliage to disguise their advance on Macbeth's castle. Coloured lithograph collector's card in a series illustrating *Macbeth*, produced to advertise a German meat extract product, *c.* 1910.

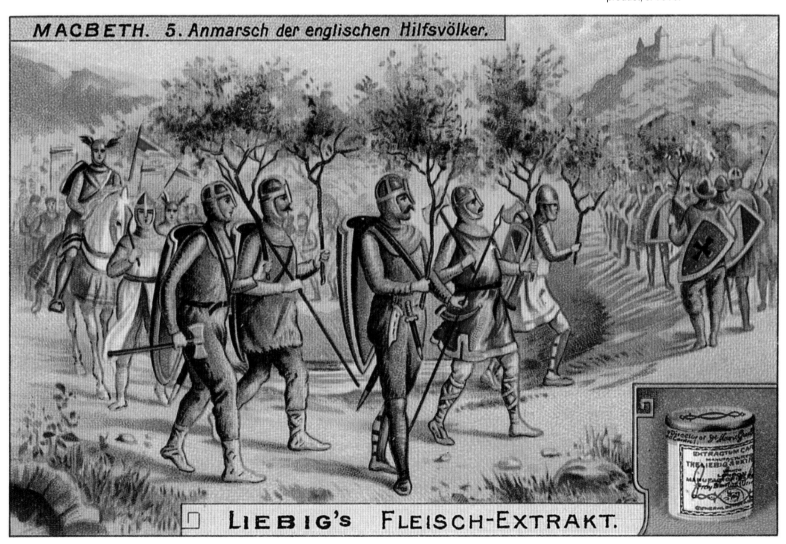

MACBETH. 5. Anmarsch der englischen Hilfsvölker.

LIEBIG's FLEISCH-EXTRAKT.

▼ **Battle of Quatre Bras**, 16 June
1815. At the beginning of the 19th
century, the majority of European
soldiers still wore brightly coloured
uniforms, but some of their comrades,
armed with rifles, were wearing more
camouflaged uniforms in shades of
green and grey.

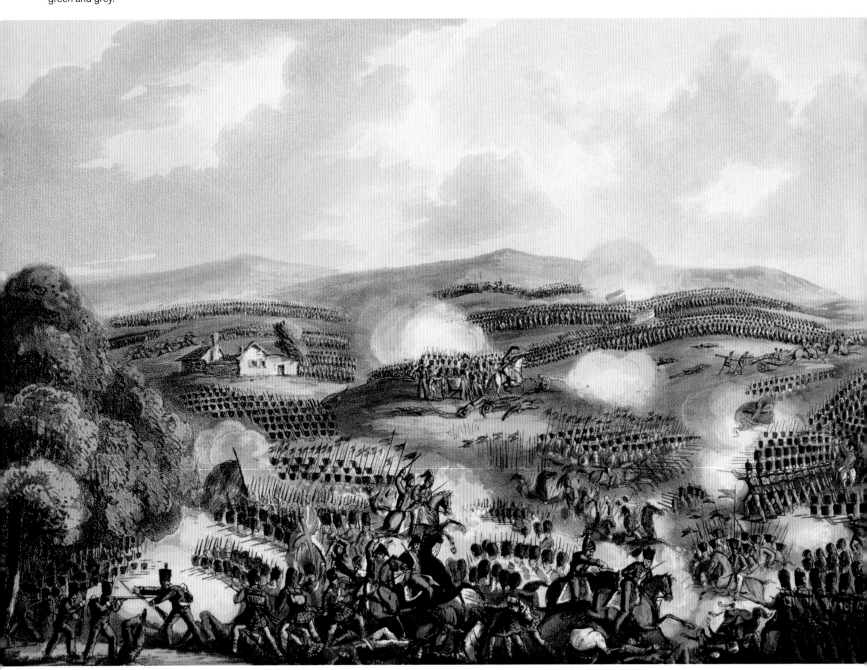

The interior of the rifle barrel was created with spiral grooves so that the bullet revolved in the air as it left the gun. Because of this it offered great improvements in accuracy and range compared with the smoothbore musket. At first, such guns were very expensive and used only by wealthy hunters, but by the 18th century they could be manufactured in sufficient numbers to be used on the battlefield. A revolution in tactics followed.

In the age of the musket in European warfare, soldiers in brightly coloured uniforms had lined up in front of each other and fired volley after volley at the enemy until one side decided it had had enough and ran. The arrival of soldiers armed with rifles changed this significantly. Skirmishers now stalked an enemy, like a hunter might, hiding themselves in long grass or behind trees and picking off enemy soldiers as they approached. In North America, by the middle of the 18th century, loose formations of riflemen were proving so effective against rigid lines of musket-bearing soldiers that the red-coated British Army created its own rifle units and clad them in green – one of the earliest forms of camouflaged uniform.

The most famous green-coated regiment in the British Army was the 95th Rifle Regiment, which had a reputation as an elite. The 95th fought in the wars against Napoleon Bonaparte's France. The men were selected for their skills at rifle shooting and the unit tended to attract more intelligent soldiers, men who could act individually, rather than just form part of a tightly drilled line. They would use their own initiative to approach the enemy, fire a single shot at an enemy officer and then disappear into the landscape. The hunting horn emblem worn on their hats and backpacks was a reference to the fact that many of these early riflemen came from a hunting background.

It was these 'Green Jackets' rather than their red-coated comrades who were the predecessors of the modern combat soldier. The romance attached to this elite force lives on today in the best-selling novels of Bernard Cornwell. His character Richard Sharpe is a green-jacketed rifleman constantly in conflict with the more regimented values of his red-coated superiors.

Central Europe has its own strong hunting tradition and it was in Austria in the middle of the 18th century that another force of sharpshooters arose. These were called *Jäger* and were recruited from foresters and huntsmen. Rather than green, they usually wore grey uniforms, made of 50 per cent undyed white wool and 50 per cent blue-dyed wool. It was this type of light grey that was later adopted by Confederate forces during the American Civil War. A study carried out by Captain Charles Hamilton Smith during the Napoleonic Wars discovered that this grey was less conspicuous than green and provided more effective camouflage at a distance of 150 yards.

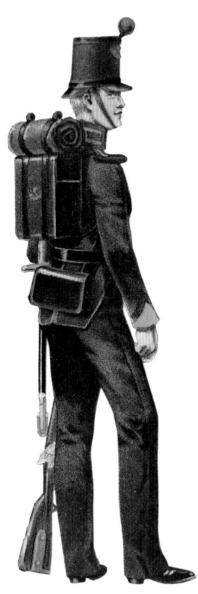

◀ **British rifleman of the 60th King's Royal Rifle Corps**, pictured in 1845. The hunting horn on his pack is a reference to the early origins of green-clad sharpshooters. The 60th King's Royal Rifle Corps was one of three infantry regiments that were amalgamated in 1966 to form the Royal Green Jackets.

▼ **Bernard Cornwell's fictional character Sharpe**, portrayed here by British actor Sean Bean in the Carlton TV series, embodies the independent qualities expected of a green-jacketed rifleman of the 95th Rifle Regiment, formed in 1800.

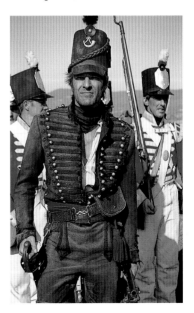

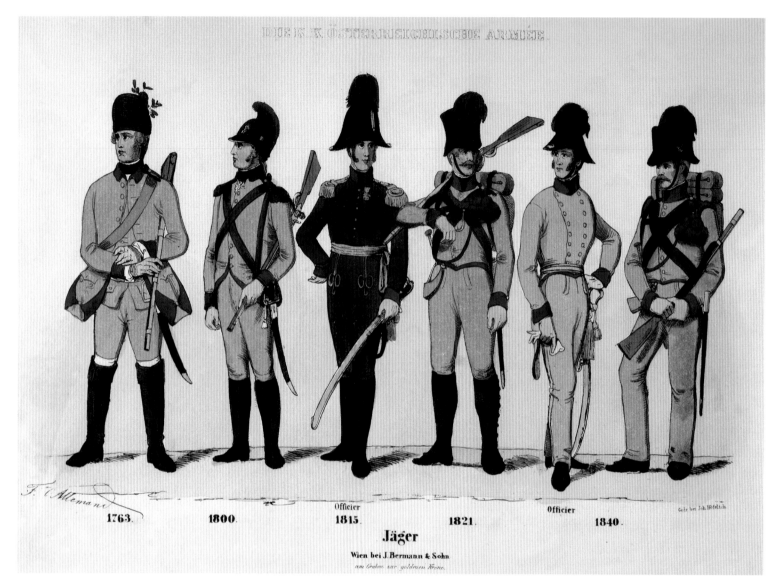

DIE K. K. ÖSTERREICHISCHE ARMÉE.

1763.   1800.   Officier 1815.   1821.   Officier 1840.

Jäger

Wien bei J. Bermann & Sohn.
am Graben zur goldenen Krone.

⬧ **Austrian *Jäger* soldiers in grey uniforms.** Early 19th-century firing tests concluded that grey was a more effective camouflage than green. It was later adopted by Confederate forces in the American Civil War. Coloured lithograph by Fritz l'Allemand, 1845.

Although green- and grey-clad riflemen had arrived on the battlefield in the 18th century, the majority of European soldiers still fought in brightly coloured uniforms for another hundred years. Despite the improved killing capacities of guns, which could fire faster and further than ever before, soldiers still liked to wear a brightly coloured, conspicuous uniform into battle – it made them feel proud and, away from the battlefield, was something in which to show off to women. But a development in India in the middle of the 19th century indicated the way forward for future military clothing and was the immediate ancestor of modern camouflage combat dress.

Dusty Soldiers

In 1846, in the Punjab region of northern India, a British officer called Harry Lumsden raised a combined unit of infantry and cavalry from tribesmen, including Sikhs, Pathans and Afghans. It was called the Corps of Guides and it became the first unit in a European army to wear a khaki uniform, consisting of loose-fitting trousers and jackets dyed a muddy colour.

Lumsden recalled that his orders specified that in order 'to get the best work out of the troops and to enable them to undertake great exertions, it was necessary that the soldier should be loosely, comfortably and suitably clad.' To meet this requirement, Lumsden bought a quantity of white cotton fabric that he then had dyed with river mud. The cloth was made into loose shirts based on the native *kurta*. The colouring was thus the product of the landscape and was more grey than brown.

Khaki is an Urdu word meaning dusty or dust-coloured, derived from the Persian word for dust or dirt, *khak*. Its potential as camouflage was soon appreciated: Major William Hodson, second-in-command of the Corps of Guides in 1848, told his brother that khaki made his soldiers 'invisible in a land of dust.'

But the new uniform confused other British soldiers and one gunner had to stop his own artillery firing at the khaki-clad troops. 'Lord! Sir,' he shouted to an officer, 'them is our mudlarks!'

A decade later, from 1857 to 1858, the Indian Mutiny raged through the subcontinent. Native soldiers rose up against the forces of the British Empire and slaughtered many European colonists. Some of the fiercest fighting took place at the height of the Indian summer and British soldiers suffered greatly in the hot weather. They abandoned their traditional European uniforms of red jackets for the lighter, unlined white clothes they wore in camp.

In the fighting, these lighter clothes became dirty and some soldiers chose to smarten them up by dyeing them with any colouring substances to hand, such as tea or curry powder, thus creating improvised khaki uniforms. In this they were no doubt also inspired by their native allies in northern India. A year later, the British Army officially recognized this new form of uniform and ordered their soldiers to wear two suits of 'khakee'.

Some British colonists were unimpressed. 'Those dreadful-looking men,' said one Englishwoman, seeing them march into town, 'must be Afghans.'

The British Army's adoption of khaki was a temporary measure. After the Indian Mutiny, it was abandoned for at least 20 years. However, there were experiments with other forms of camouflage, such as a grey-brown tweed jacket designed for fighting against the Ashanti in West Africa in 1873. In the 1879 war against the Zulus, British soldiers stained their white sun helmets and belts with tea.

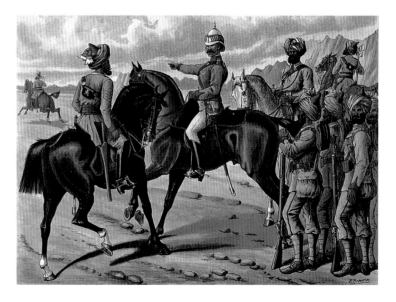

☑ **The Corps of Guides**, raised in northern India by Harry Lumsden in 1846, was the first unit in the British Army to wear khaki. Illustration by Richard Simkin, *c.* 1885.

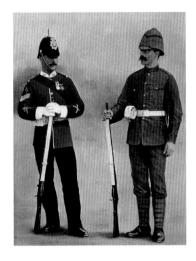

The two styles of British Army uniform in 1900, worn by a Colour-Sergeant and Private of the Gloucester Regiment. Just two years later khaki had been accepted for home service too, relegating the red jacket to a purely ceremonial role.

Sealed pattern khaki tunic of 1902, the year in which khaki became the official uniform of the British Army for home and overseas service. A sealed pattern uniform is one approved by the Army Board of Ordnance, sealed with wax, and thus established as the definitive pattern for that item of clothing.

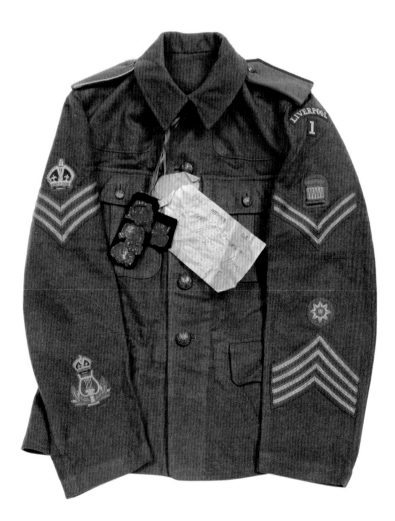

Eventually, it was decided that nothing improved upon the original khaki and in 1896 it was officially accepted into the British Army for all overseas service. In 1902, khaki finally displaced scarlet by becoming the official uniform colour of the British Army at home and abroad.

Other modern armies were yet to be convinced by the use of khaki and stuck to their traditional colours. Only in the US, perhaps as a result of its own colonial war in the Philippines, did khaki also become the official combat uniform colour in 1902. Even at the outset of the First World War in 1914, some countries still insisted on fighting in uniforms of their national colours. The French marched to war on the Western Front in blue jackets and red trousers. But the devastating effect of modern warfare soon saw a dulling down of these colours into 'horizon blue'. In other armies, grey became the most common alternative to khaki for combat clothes.

Camouflage of Artillery and Fortifications

There is tantalizing evidence that, long before the use of the word 'camouflage' in the First World War, the British Army was employing its principles to disguise coastal gun emplacements. Lieutenant-General Andrew Clarke was the Inspector-General of Fortifications in 1886 when he made the following report to the War Office in London. 'Fortified ports will not in future be marked by batteries conspicuously frowning, or granite casemated forts with tiers of guns rivalling rows of targets in regularity and clearness of definition. On the contrary, defences, if skilfully disguised, will be indistinguishable from the ground in which they stand, and while they retain all the advantages of defence, will offer no mark for an enemy's fire.' As an example he cited the new port defences in Singapore, which he declared 'practically invisible from the sea'.

That paint was also used to achieve these results was indicated by a report to the War Office in the same year on the defences of Malta. It mentioned a battery on the sea front and recommended that 'if the concrete were coloured and the gun distempered, the battery would be hard to make out.' Distemper is a kind of whitewash whose matt finish dulled the shine of the gun barrels.

A letter from Josephine Richardson published in *The Times* in 1939 suggested that far more elaborate camouflage schemes had been in use on home coastal gun emplacements in 1890. She recalled that Colonel John Booth Richardson had 'the forts looking out to sea painted in broad reds, greens and yellows'. She claimed this was the first use of military camouflage and said she had accompanied her father in a boat to view the schemes. How effective they were remains uncertain. 'A poor sailor and very short-sighted,' she wrote, 'I was only too ready to answer "no" when asked whether the forts were distinguishable.'

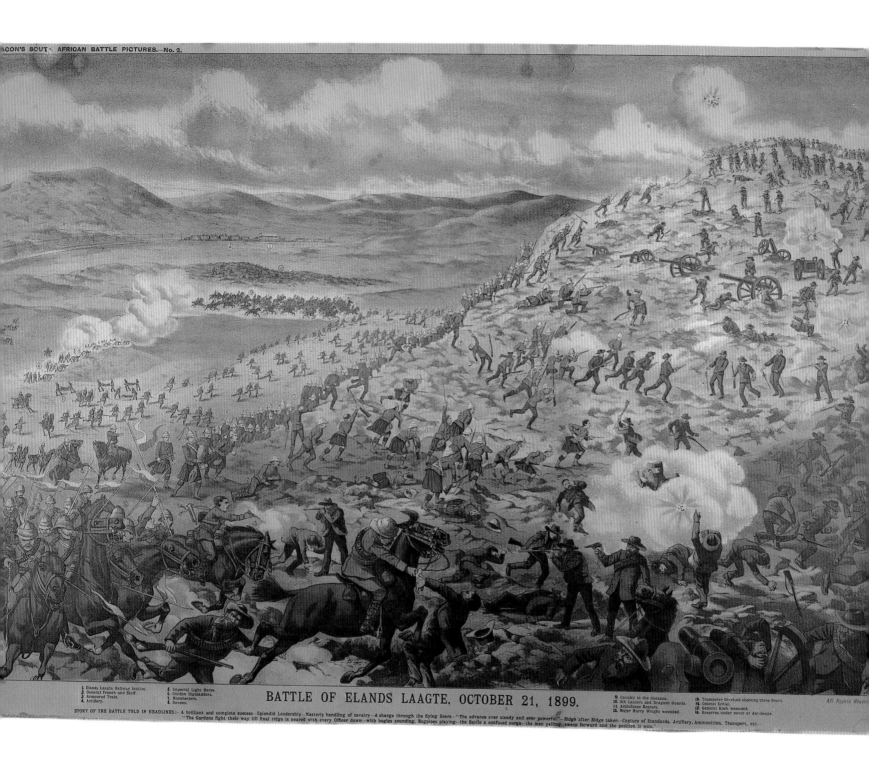

BATTLE OF ELANDS LAAGTE, OCTOBER 21, 1899.

▲ **The Battle of Elandslaagte, 21 October 1899**. Unusually for a poster of the time, this illustration depicts British troops in khaki jackets; most popular illustrations continued to show the British Army clad in the scarlet uniforms much loved by the Victorian public.

Hunting and Camouflage

Hunters have always been skilled *camoufleurs*. Their closeness to nature means they know a great deal about how animals disguise themselves. Frequently, they celebrate their affinity with nature by wearing feathers or furs which themselves act as a form of camouflage.

The inventiveness of hunters has produced a wide variety of decoys and disguises, but perhaps the most extraordinary form of hunting camouflage is the ghillie suit. Originally devised by Scottish gamekeepers, or ghillies, as a kind of portable hide-out, the idea is to cover the hunter in dozens of ragged strips of cloth attached to netting worn over his usual hunting clothes. The ragged strips of material break up the hunter's silhouette and merge with the surrounding foliage. The suit frequently incorporates padding too as it may be worn for a long time while the hunter remains still, waiting for his prey.

Ghillie suits have long been adapted by the military as perfect camouflage for snipers. Most military snipers take the time to make their own personalized ghillie suits, adapted to the particular environment they are serving in. A variant of the ghillie suit that uses strips of heat-conductive

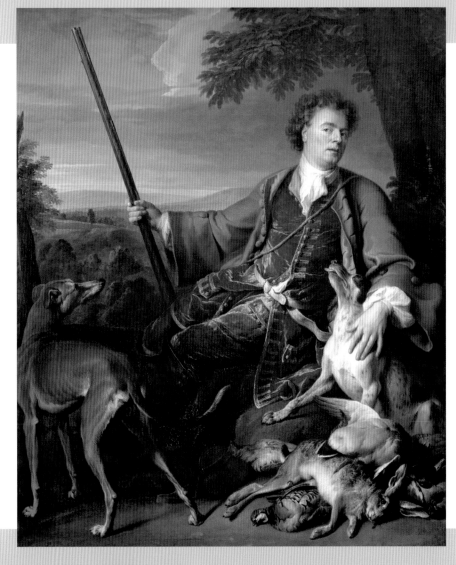

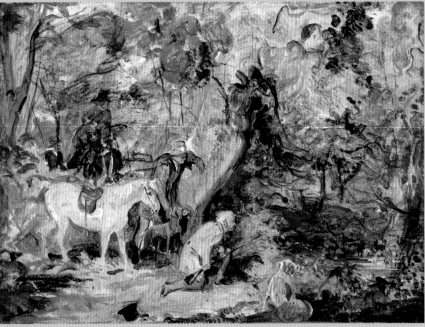

▲ **François Desportes, *Self-Portrait as a Hunter*, 1699.** The artist wears a loose brown hunting jacket to cover up his bright civilian clothing.

◄ **Sketch for *Foresters Stalking Deer* by John Frederick Lewis.** The use of rifles from the 16th century onwards gave hunters greater range and accuracy. When combined with camouflage hunting shirts, as depicted in this mid-19th-century sketch, they gave hunters a huge advantage over their quarry.

▶ **Emperor Franz Josef of Austria** was a keen hunter and is portrayed here wearing a *Jäger* grey hunting jacket. Postcard of 1908.

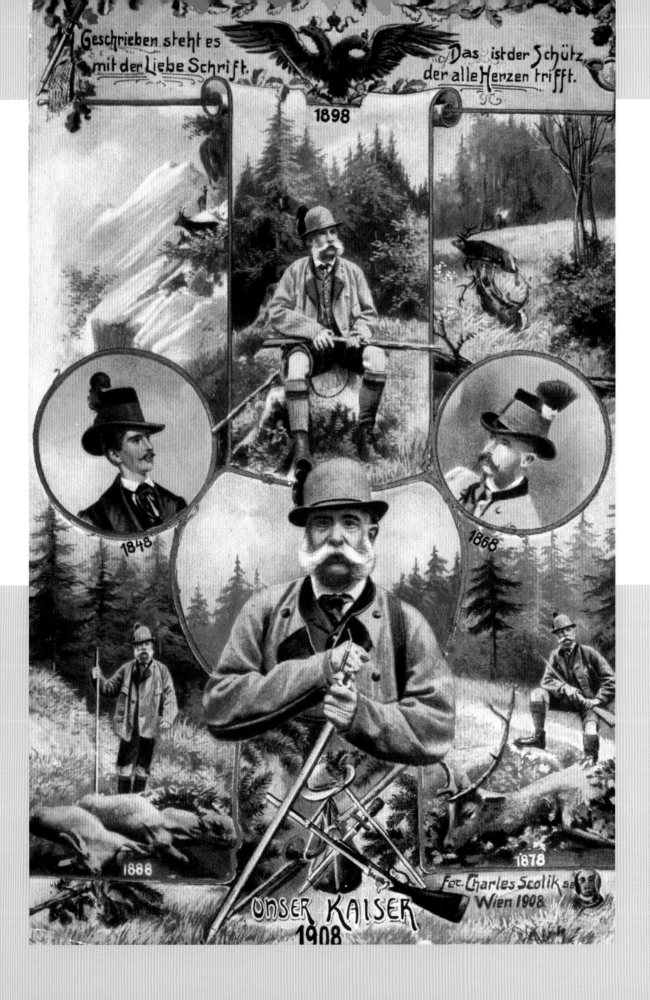

Geschrieben steht es mit der Liebe Schrift.

Das ist der Schütz der alle Herzen trifft.

1898

1848

1868

1888

1878

Fec. Charles Scolik sa. Wien 1908

UNSER KAISER 1908

material to disperse the soldier's body heat has even been experimented with as a means of thwarting detection by thermal imaging devices.

Hunting has always provided inspiration for military camouflage. In the early 1960s, when camouflage combat dress had fallen out of official favour in the US Army, some American military advisors in Vietnam wore duck-hunting camouflage bought from civilian suppliers. Hunters are continually searching for the perfect camouflage. In 1986 American hunter Bill Jordan devised a new range of highly naturalistic camouflage patterns by overlaying images of leaves, twigs and bark. These create a three-dimensional effect that blends in with a range of terrains and is highly distinctive to Jordan's range of clothing sold under the label Realtree.

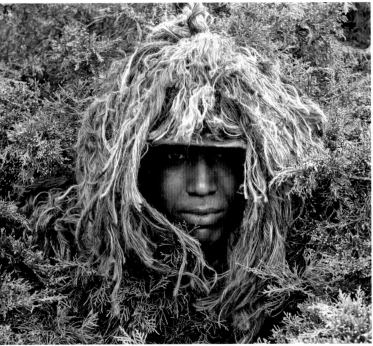

◭ **A ghillie suit** enables a US soldier to blend into the terrain during a training mission in Germany, 2004.

◪ **A knitted hat studded with branches** helps camouflage this member of the Eagle Hunt Club in Poland. Wearing such foliage or feathers in a hat is an enduring hunting tradition that was also one of the very earliest forms of camouflage.

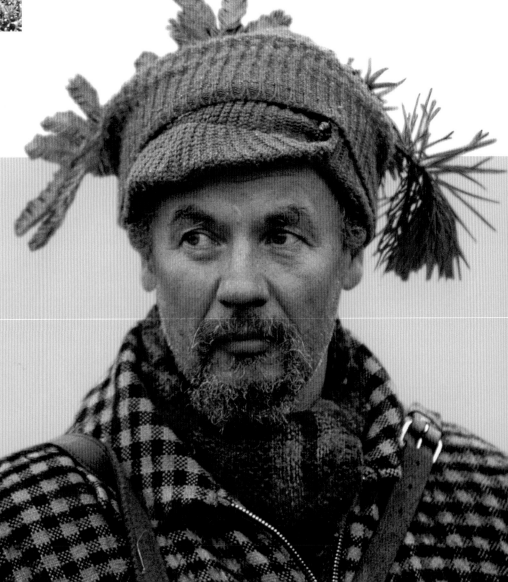

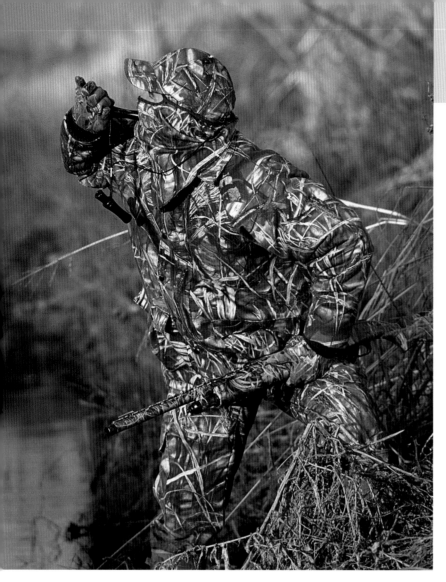

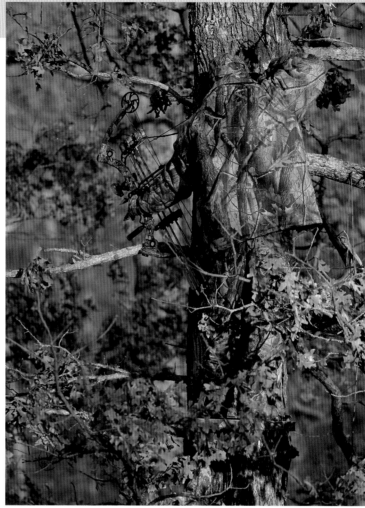

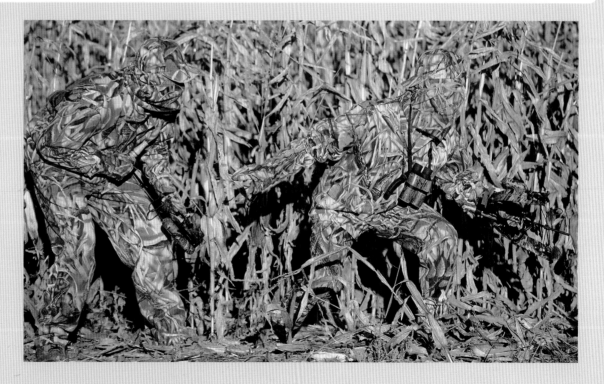

△ ▷ **American hunters wearing 'Realtree' camouflage patterns.** These excellent designs combine images of twigs and leaves with the bark of a tree to produce highly specific and effective camouflage for contemporary hunters in a range of different landscape settings. The company was founded by Bill Jordan in 1986.

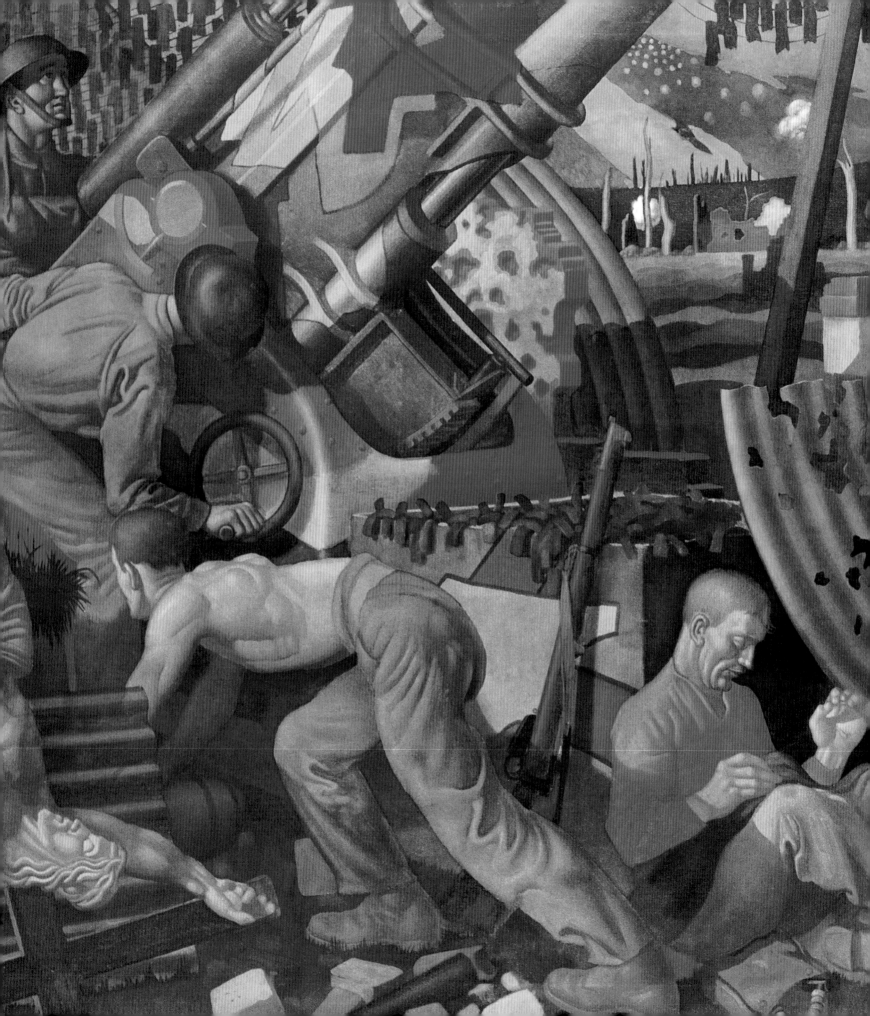

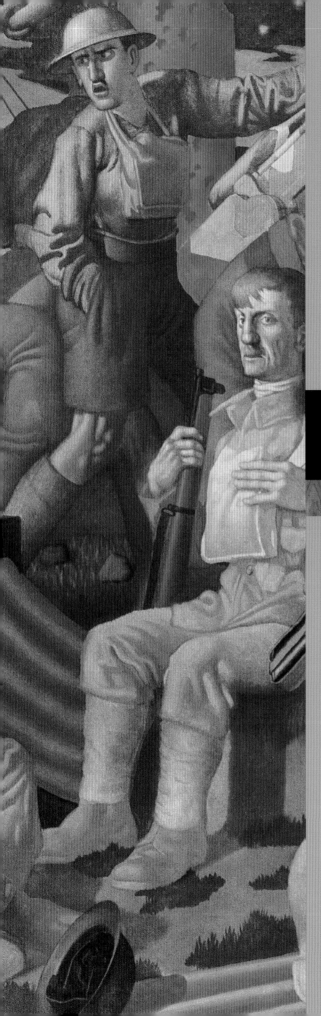

Defeating the Eye in the Sky
Camouflage in the First World War

With the outbreak of the First World War, the new threat of aerial reconnaissance spurred new creativity in the military arts of disguise. Camouflage units were formed by all sides. Their members, often operating at the front, experimented with bold disruptive patterns on guns, tanks and aircraft. Most striking of all were the Dazzle designs applied to ships, which resembled floating Cubist paintings.

Defeating the Eye in the Sky
Camouflage in the First World War

Previous page: *Heavy Artillery*, oil on canvas, Colin Gill, 1919 (detail). A group of British soldiers man a heavy artillery position. Three of them are engaged in aiming and preparing to fire a heavy gun painted with a colourful disruptive pattern.

▽ **The construction of a hidden gun emplacement** as revealed in pages from a watercolour sketchbook by French *camoufleur* Raymond Monbiot, July 1917.

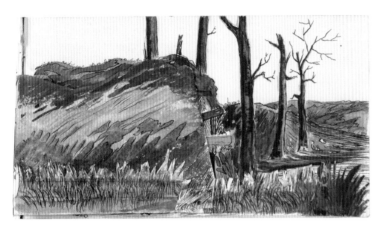

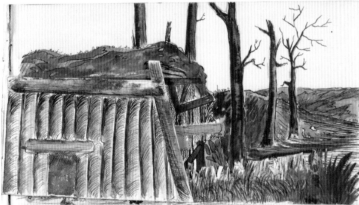

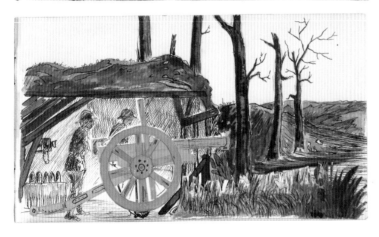

The birth of modern camouflage was a direct consequence of the invention of the aeroplane. Aircraft were initially used in the First World War for aerial reconnaissance. Their task was to spot enemy positions and note the artillery, soldiers and vehicles gathered there. With this information, they could instruct their own artillery to direct fire at these targets. This process led to a deadly game of hide-and-seek in which each side tried to disguise any build-up of artillery and soldiers and so retain the advantage of surprise before any major offensive. Camouflage now became a major factor in this combat of deception.

The first efforts at camouflage took the form of either painting big guns or covering them with painted tarpaulins or netting. The colours initially chosen were greens or browns to merge with the background, but it was soon discovered that the use of black or dark colours painted next to lighter colours had the effect of visually breaking up the shape of guns and other equipment when seen from above. This was the first use of disruptive pattern in a military context.

With direct human observation from the ground supplanted by aerial photography in black and white, contrast and shape came to matter more than colour. This liberated camouflage artists who could now use all kinds of bright colours, just so long as they broke up the form of the guns they were painting with contrasting random shapes in light and dark tones. From 1916, when tanks first came into operational use, these were also painted in camouflage schemes. Seeing these lumbering monsters splashed with bright colours proved an irresistible subject for some frontline artists. Futurist artist C.R.W. Nevinson painted an especially menacing tank in 1917, daubed with green, black and red stripes.

French and British Artists

France led the way in the employment of camouflage artists to disguise weaponry in the First World War. British Army camouflage expert Solomon J. Solomon acknowledged this debt: 'not until a year and a half after the outbreak of war,' he wrote, 'and a year after [camouflage] was to some extent adopted by the French, did we follow their lead.'

In a wartime issue of British news magazine *The Sphere* of 3 August 1918, Lucien-Victor Guirand de Scévola, a Parisian portraitist serving with the artillery at Toul in 1914, was credited with being the first artist to camouflage artillery. He was followed by a number of French artists, including Eugène Corbin, Jean-Louis Forain, Abel Truchet, Joseph Pinchon and Marcel Bain, who contributed their talents to disguising big guns. They went on to serve in specialist camouflage sections that were eventually attached to each army in the field.

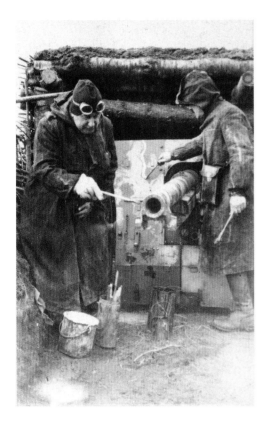

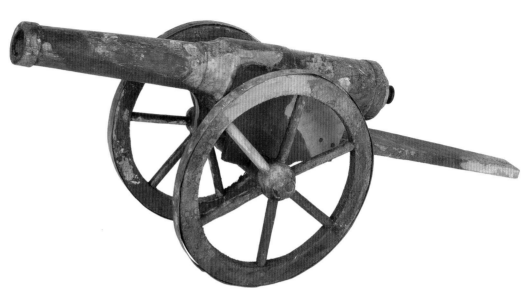

△ **Camouflage artists** painting a gun on the Western Front. On the left is the French painter and illustrator Jean-Louis Forain.

◪ **Model gun** painted in disruptive pattern camouflage by French *camoufleur* Eugène Corbin.

▶ **A Tank**, oil painting by C.R.W. Nevinson, 1917. Nevinson's earlier war art was heavily influenced by Futurism and sought to portray the dynamic beauty of modern warfare. But his paintings from 1915 depict the grim reality of battle of the Western Front.

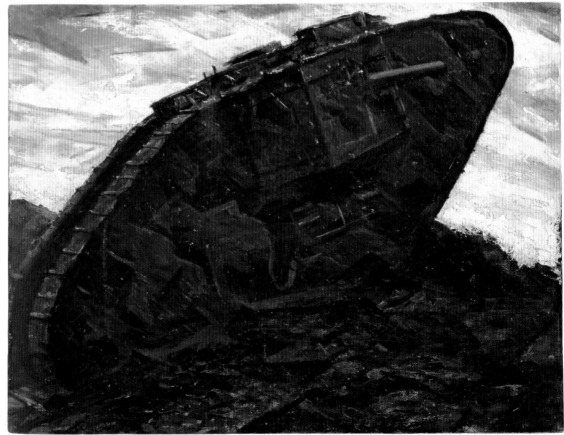

De Scévola was rapidly promoted from private to captain and by the end of the war oversaw numerous workshops along the Western Front employing 1,200 men and 8,000 women. Even in the midst of warfare, he was reportedly something of a dandy who liked always to be elegantly dressed with white kid gloves.

Being a camouflage artist – a *camoufleur* – could be a dangerous business and *The Sphere* quoted a roll of honour of French artist casualties that listed 15 dead. Many more were wounded. They included: 'the painters Hoffner and Perille, the scene-painter André Mare, Paul Verlet, son of the celebrated sculptor, hit by a bullet full in the chest in the course of a reconnaissance, and the humorous designer Falke, who saw his right hand shot through because he would, at fifty yards from the enemy, go out of the trench a second time in order to put the finishing touch to a camouflage which was considered unfinished.'

The Sphere explored the derivation of the word 'camouflage' and tracked it back to 17th-century France when the word 'camouflet' meant a puff of smoke blown into the face of someone with the malicious intent of blinding and confusing them. Beyond that, it could be traced to the Walloon words 'foumer', to smoke, and 'cafouma', a puff of smoke. Another derivation is the French verb 'camoufler', meaning to make up for the stage.

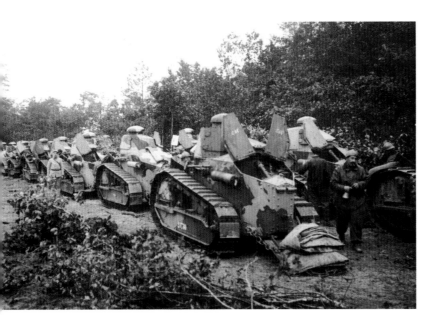

◤ **Camouflage French Renault FT-17 tanks**, 1918. This lightweight tank went into mass production towards the end of the war, and was widely used by the French and the Americans.

▶ **Disguising a British field gun** with paint and netting on the Western Front. Illustration published in *The Sphere*, August 1918, from a painting by S. Ugo.

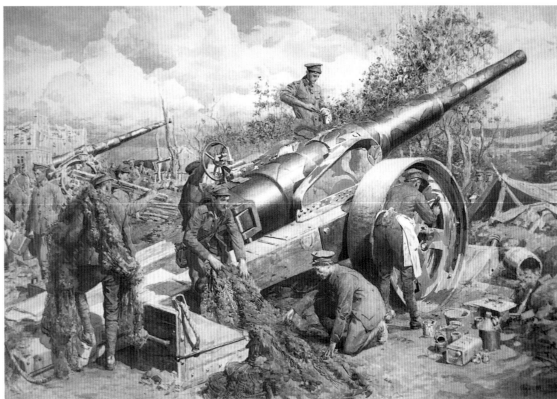

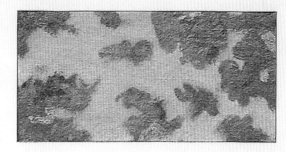

Secteur de Champagne.

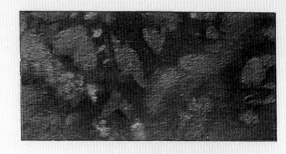

Secteur de l'Aisne (bois).

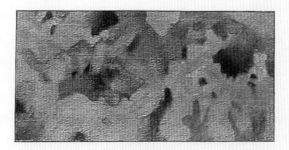

Secteur du Santerre, au printemps.

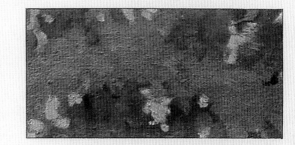

Secteur de Lorraine.

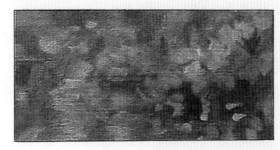

Secteur des Flandres.

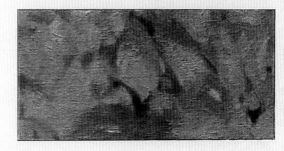

Secteur de l'Oise.

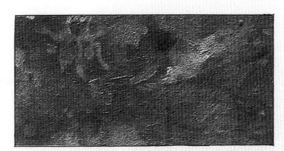

Secteur des Vosges.

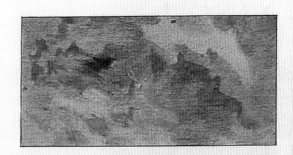

Chemin des Dames.

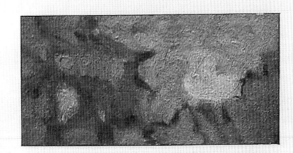

Secteur de Verdun.

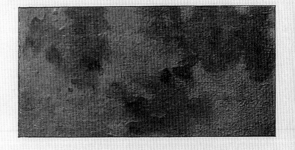

Secteur de l'Argonne.

UNE CARTE D'ECHANTILLONS DU CAMOUFLAGE. — Les secteurs du front.

Chacun de ces échantillons donne la tonalité générale du terrain d'un secteur et indique les nuances et dispositions à adopter pour l'imitation en toile peinte de ce terrain.

◨ **Colour chart** produced by French *camoufleurs* to show the general tonality of the terrain along different sections of the French Western Front. Such charts were used as colour guides for the painting of camouflage fabric and screens. This example is from an article in *L'Illustration*, 1920.

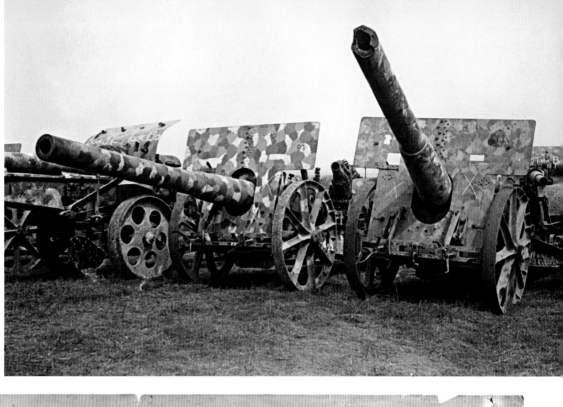

▶ **Camouflaged German field artillery** captured by Australian and Canadian Divisions during the second Battle of the Somme, August 1918.

▽ **British War Office design** suggesting a camouflage painting scheme for field artillery.

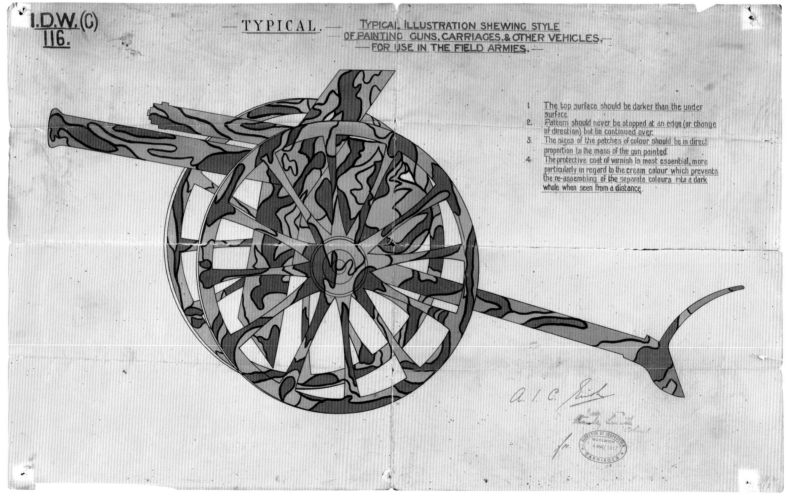

I.D.W.(C) 116.

— TYPICAL. — TYPICAL ILLUSTRATION SHEWING STYLE OF PAINTING GUNS, CARRIAGES, & OTHER VEHICLES, — FOR USE IN THE FIELD ARMIES.

1. The top surface should be darker than the under surface.
2. Pattern should never be stopped at an edge (or change of direction) but be continued over.
3. The sizes of the patches of colour should be in direct proportion to the mass of the gun painted.
4. The protective coat of varnish is most essential, more particularly in regard to the cream colour which prevents the re-assembling of the separate colours into a dark whole when seen from a distance.

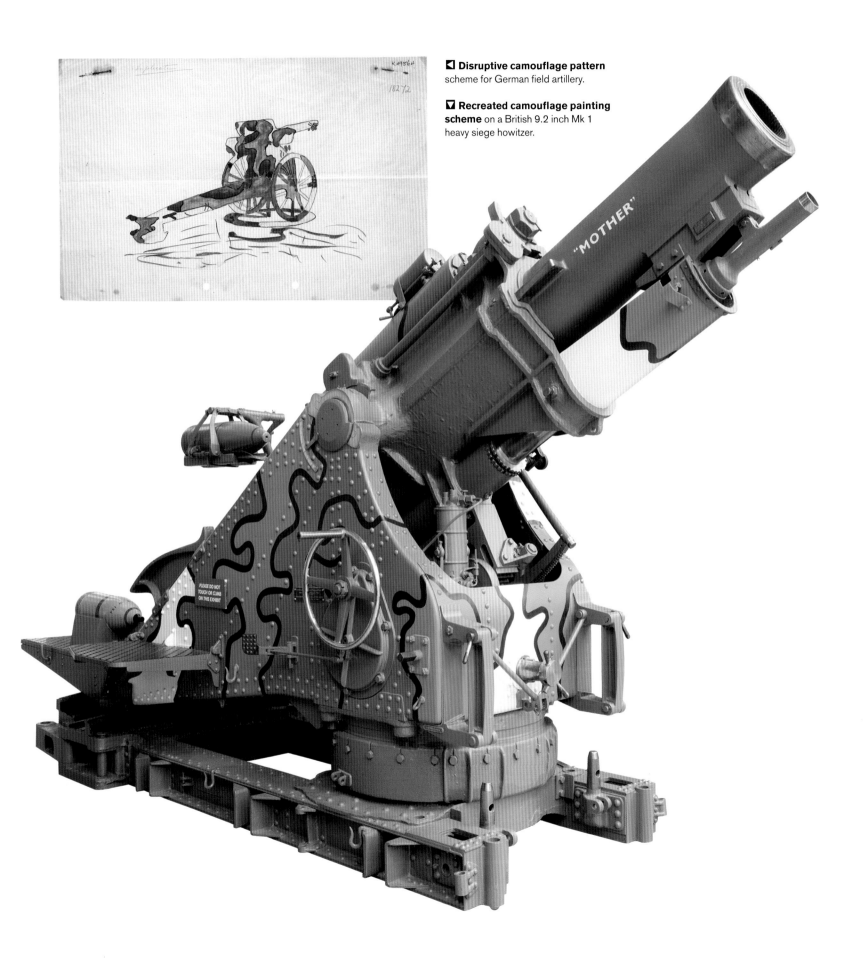

◀ **Disruptive camouflage pattern**
scheme for German field artillery.

▼ **Recreated camouflage painting
scheme** on a British 9.2 inch Mk 1
heavy siege howitzer.

"MOTHER"

PLEASE DO NOT
TOUCH OR CLIMB
ON THIS EXHIBIT

At first, the British were confident that khaki was sufficient disguise for military equipment, but they took note of French developments in disruptive pattern schemes, and by 1916 had raised their own camouflage section. It was commanded by Lieutenant-Colonel Francis Wyatt of the Royal Engineers and included many prominent artists. A key advisor was Solomon J. Solomon, an artist who had enjoyed precocious success in his twenties and remained a popular illustrator. Now in his fifties, he proved a dynamic proponent of the importance of camouflage and believed that being an artist was an essential qualification to carrying it out effectively.

'The *camoufleur* is, of course, an artist,' he wrote, 'preferably one who paints or sculpts imaginative subjects, with some deductive faculties. He must leave no clues for the detective on the other side in what he designs or executes, and he must above all things be resourceful. But his imagination and inventiveness should have free play.'

Alongside Solomon worked the avant-garde sculptor Leon Underwood, who created a series of beautiful sketches showing the kind of work he carried out. Ernest Shepard, who served as an officer in the Royal Artillery on the Western Front, made a study of his camouflaged gun position during the Battle of the Somme in August 1916. Shepard was later to become famous as the illustrator of A.A. Milne's series of children's books about Winnie the Pooh.

Solomon was aware that some soldiers considered the use of camouflage as unchivalrous, but those critics can 'never have visualized the conditions of modern war...for the side which neglects it will be unduly exposed to the onslaught of an adversary who will be concealed, and whose whereabouts cannot be detected.' Far from being a mere sideshow, Solomon argued that an effective understanding of camouflage lay at the very heart of winning a modern war.

Solomon's camouflage unit was attached to the Royal Engineers in Wimereux, France. Under the disguised name of the 'Special Works Park', it ran several workshops to produce camouflage materials. A camouflage school was also set up in London, in Kensington Gardens, to instruct commanding officers. By the end of the war, the Special Works Park in Wimereux could lay claim to having produced one million square yards of painted canvas, over four million yards of scrim, six million yards of wire netting and seven million square yards of fish netting, all of which was used in camouflage projects.

The British summarized their experience in a 29-page booklet published in March 1918 called *The Principles and Practice of Camouflage*. 'The chief opponent to be overcome,' said the booklet, 'is the expert, who, with the advantages of time and undisturbed concentration which are lacking to the aeroplane observer, is able

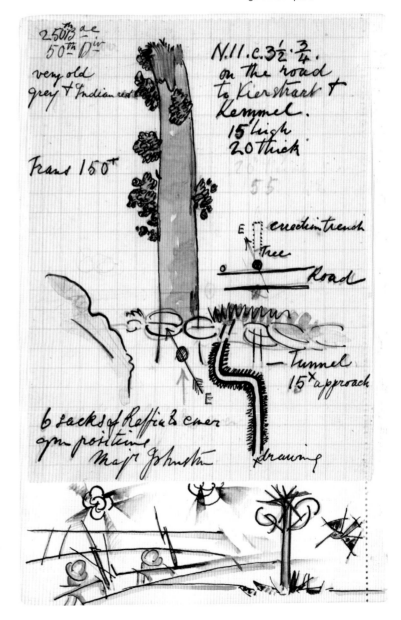

▽ **Page from a sketchbook by Leon Underwood** recording details of military observation posts disguised as trees. Underwood worked as a camouflage artist for the British on the Western Front. Before the war, he was an avant-garde sculptor.

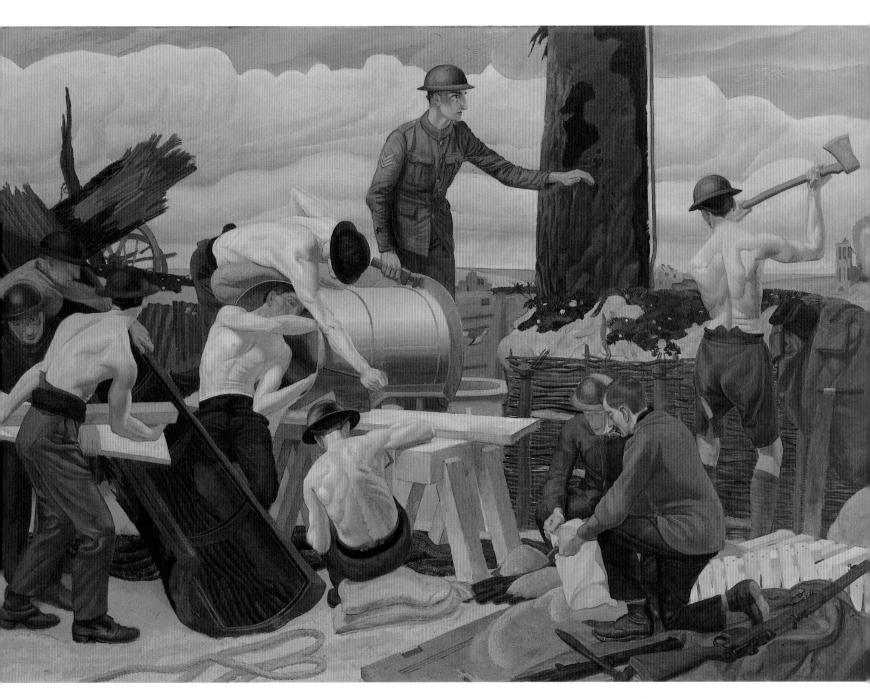

▲ *Erecting a Camouflage Tree*,
oil painting by Leon Underwood, 1919.
Such fake trees, built around a hollow
metal cylinder, were used by military
observers to watch enemy troop
movements. Unlike here, they would
generally be constructed under cover
of darkness.

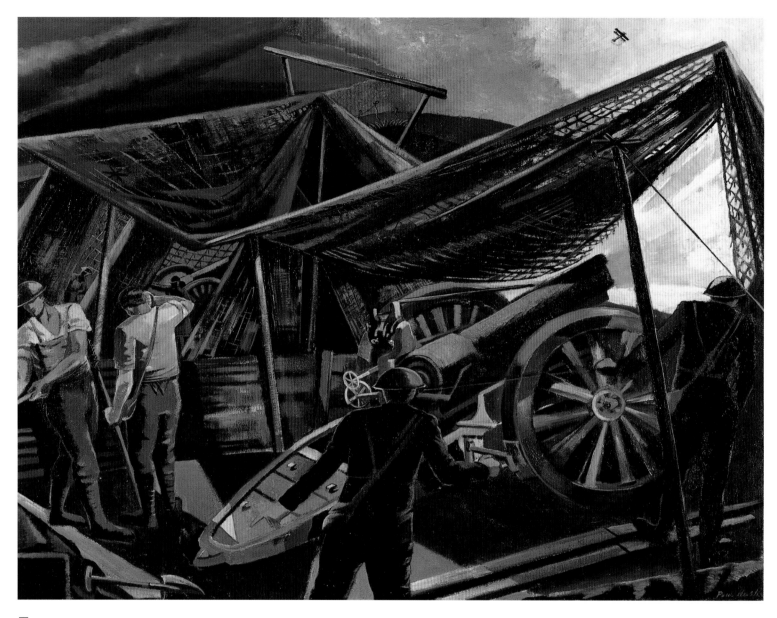

◤ *A Howitzer Firing*, oil painting by Paul Nash, 1918. Four British artillerymen stand beneath a canopy of camouflage netting as they fire a howitzer. The men on the left are shielding themselves from the muzzle flash.

to interpret what is recorded on photographs. The camera is a most accurate witness, and a photograph will always record something. The art of camouflage lies in conveying a misleading impression as to what that something means.'

Among the biggest giveaways were the disturbance of soil and vegetation, tracks left by vehicles, the shadows of military objects, and blast marks left by firing guns. It was in this world of detail photographed from above that much camouflage activity functioned. All spoil from digging was to be concealed, military vehicles were to be kept to single-line tracks placed near hedges or trees, while military equipment was to be placed close to other bigger shadow-casting objects such as hedges and houses. The absence of blast marks indicated an area was unoccupied, and this was best achieved by firing guns over bare earth or a road, but faked blast marks, on grass, could be used to deceive observers.

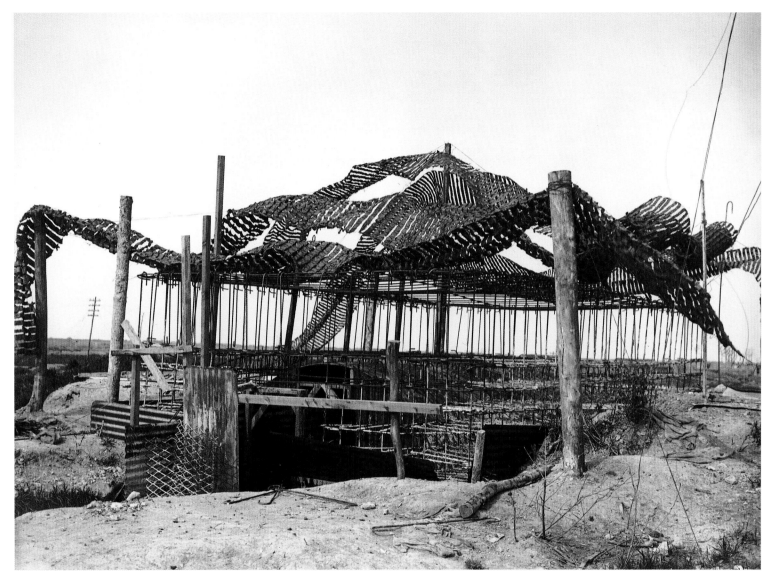

⬟ **Camouflage netting** raised on a framework over an incomplete dugout at Ypres.

Fish netting or wire netting covered with canvas or local foliage were the most widely used camouflage materials, though it was important to keep such covers away from the muzzles of firing guns. 'Many disastrous fires have been caused by neglect of this precaution,' advised *The Principles and Practice of Camouflage*, 'particularly in the case of heavy howitzers which, having recoiled bodily after coming into action for the first time, have been fired again without readjustment of the opening in the camouflage.' The use of local foliage to cover a position for any length of time was not a good idea as once it turned brown it became easily distinguishable from the surrounding environment.

The most effective camouflage for artillery was to treat a whole area as one unit. For example, an entire fake field could be created that conformed to the usual agricultural boundaries of the area and yet beneath its netting were a number of howitzers.

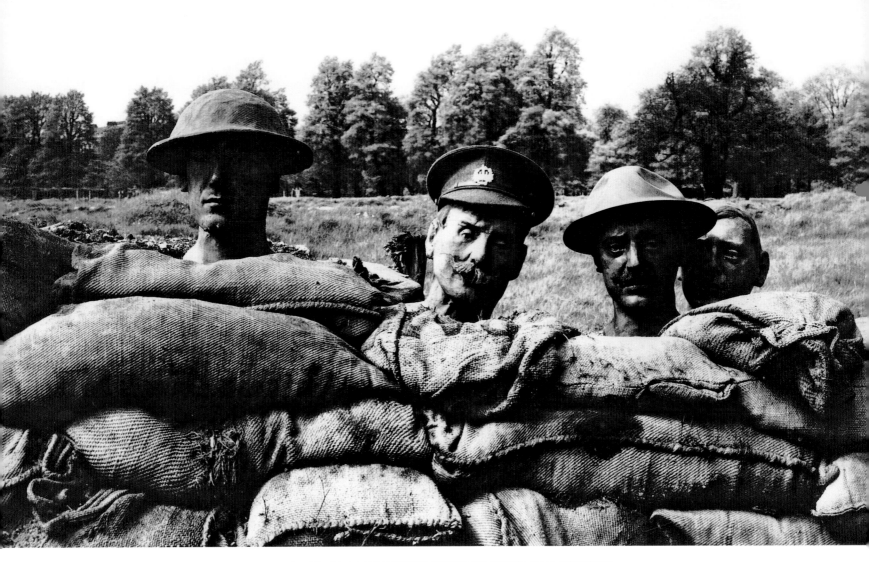

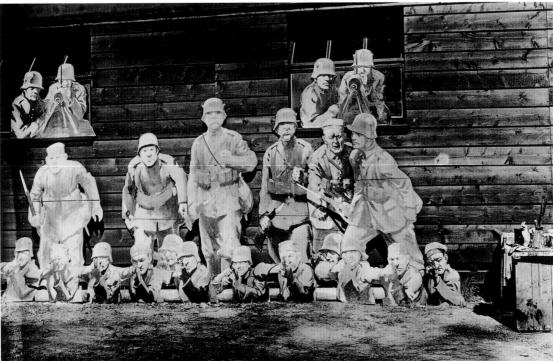

◁ ◩ **British camouflage devices** during the First World War included papier-mâché heads (above) intended to deceive enemy snipers, and board figures (left), many depicting Germans, that were intended to mislead the enemy and disguise attacks. These photographs were taken at the British Camouflage School based in Kensington Gardens, London.

Much of the British camouflage booklet is devoted to hiding weaponry, but some is designed to protect soldiers. Fake figures made of board were recommended for what were termed 'Chinese Attacks'. The figures were to be raised behind smoke screens above trenches a few minutes before Zero Hour on one or both flanks of an attack in an effort to draw fire away from the real advance.

Observation posts were sometimes built inside fake trees and equipped with periscopes to watch enemy troop movements (see pages 60–61). Ideally, these were built inside close copies of existing trees, the real ones being removed and replaced during the night. Building fake trees was a complex and laborious process, however, and was discouraged 'as their construction and erection involve a considerable amount of skilled labour which can ill be spared.'

A French 78-page supplement, *Le Camouflage aux Armées*, published in the French journal *La Guerre Documentée* around 1920, recorded other elaborate and imaginative camouflage schemes. Among these were a sniper post hidden beneath a false water-filled crater and an observation post inside a dummy dead horse.

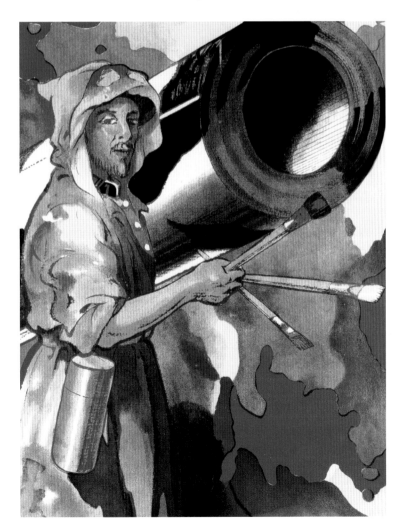

◀ **French *camoufleur*** painting a gun barrel. Illustration from *La Guerre et les Artistes*, published in Paris *c*. 1920.

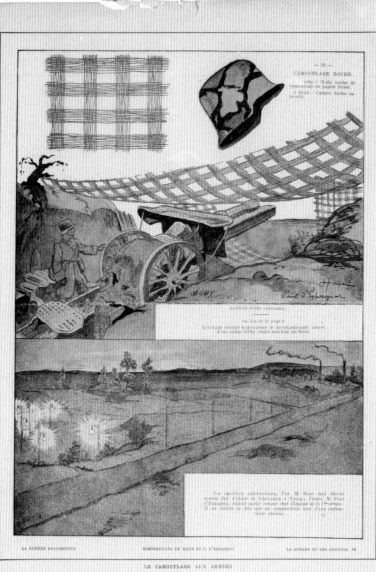

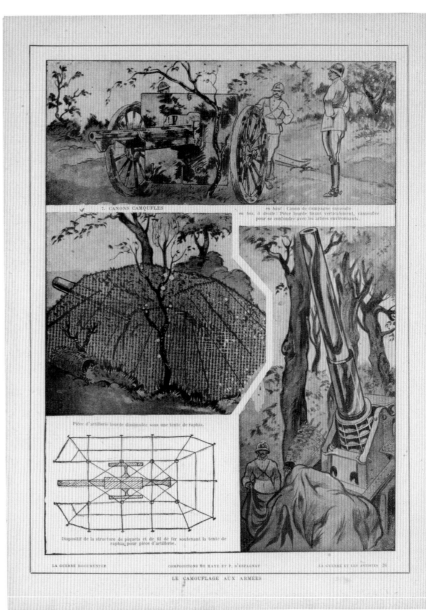

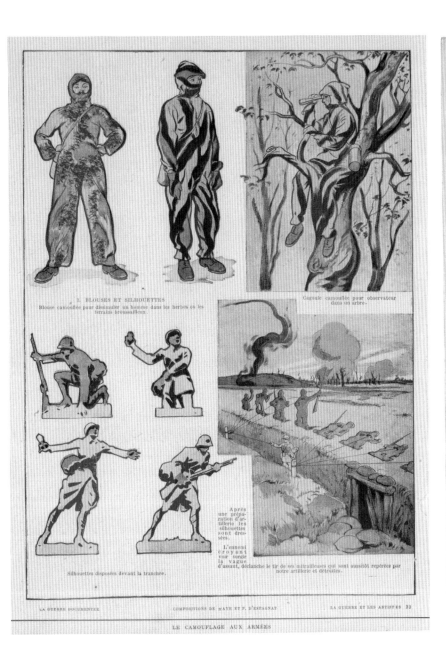

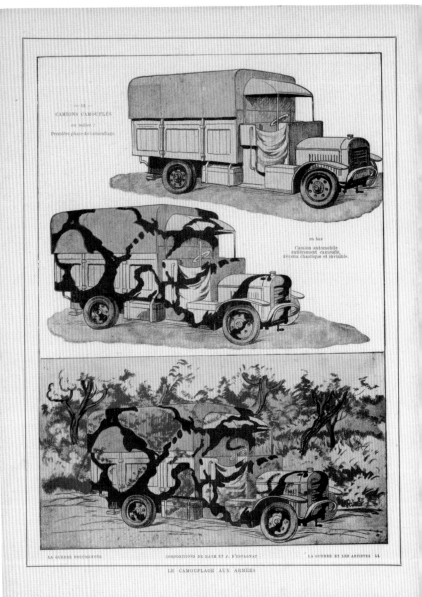

△ Pages from *La Guerre et les Artistes*, published in volume IV of *La Guerre Documentée*, Paris c. 1920, with illustrations by De Haye and P. d'Espagnat. Note the camouflage overalls for use by snipers and observers (this page, left) and the example of how disruptive pattern painting disguises a truck (this page, right).

◹ Disguised German anti-aircraft gun post. The soldiers have attached leaves and foliage to their helmets to aid their concealment.

◹ ◹ Extraordinary 3-D pattern painted on the fuselage of a British Sopwith Camel, plus hypnotic spiral on its landing wheels that made it difficult to judge their direction. Bold and colourful disruptive patterns could – and on aircraft frequently did – slip from being functional camouflage to conspicuous display.

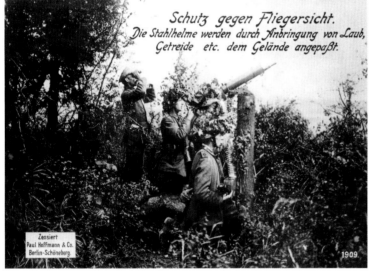

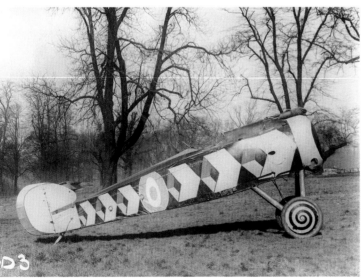

Secrets of German Camouflage

The German army also recruited artists to disguise their weaponry. The most famous of these was Franz Marc, an Expressionist painter who served initially as a cavalryman. He wrote a revealing letter to his wife in February 1916 in which he told of the creative pleasure he derived from painting military tarpaulins by adapting the styles of great modern painters.

'The business has a totally practical purpose,' said Marc, 'to hide artillery emplacements from airborne spotters and photography by covering them with tarpaulins painted in roughly pointillistic designs in the manner of bright natural camouflage. The distances which one has to reckon with are enormous – from an average height of 2000 metres – your enemy aircraft never flies much lower than that.... I am curious what effect the "Kandinskys" will have at 2000 metres. The nine tarpaulins chart a development "from Manet to Kandinsky".'

A month later, Marc returned to the cavalry and was killed near Verdun.

Disruptive patterns were the best method of camouflaging moving objects that could not easily be made to merge into a constantly shifting background. This was especially true of aircraft, where the Germans took disruptive pattern to a new level of military decoration by covering their planes in brightly coloured patterns – most notably the 'lozenge' type. All of the wing surfaces and all or some of the fuselage of the aircraft were covered in fantastic hexagonal or polygonal shapes in a riot of garish colours, with the underside in lighter colours than the upper areas.

Sometimes these patterns were printed on material fixed to the aircraft during manufacture, or they could be hand-painted in the field. Some lozenge-patterned fabrics were printed in as many as four or five separate colours. Although intended to conceal, some of these highly colourful schemes soon became a new form of heraldry by which self-proclaimed knights of the sky could show off their killing talents and achieve personal renown.

The 'Red' Baron Manfred von Richthofen and his 'Flying Circus' were the most famous of these colourful air aces – painting their planes in individual and often colourful styles (although not using the lozenge pattern). It was the beginning of a paradoxical process by which pattern that began as camouflage became a form of conspicuous insignia intended to intimidate an enemy – a form of display rather than concealment.

Solomon J. Solomon believed the Germans were far more advanced in the art of large position camouflage than the Allies and this was already in practice at the beginning of the war. He later published photographic evidence showing sophisticated earth-covered German anti-aircraft shelters in use as early as the summer of 1914. He called this 'Strategic Camouflage', and was furious with British commanders for not having recognized it earlier. Writing in 1920, he admitted that 'No British or French expert reader [of reconnaissance photographs] from the beginning of the war until 1918 had reason to suspect the existence of a German method of concealment which differed materially from our own, or was so much more extensive.' However, 'The evidence of German methods was laid before the authorities early in March 1918,' when 'it was not only doubted, but was officially repudiated, not once but again and again, till the end of the war...'.

Solomon then quoted General Erich Ludendorff's *My War Memories 1914–1918* in which the German commander made reference to forty or fifty divisions of German soldiers being crowded into elaborate systems of disguised anti-aircraft shelters. Ludendorff also laid claim to hiding whole railway transport networks just behind the frontline.

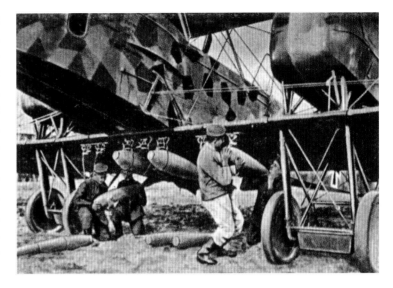

▲ **Loading a German bomber** camouflaged in 'lozenge' pattern fabric. Photograph from *Der Weltkrieg*, 1918.

▼ **German multi-coloured camouflage fabric** in 'lozenge' pattern for covering an aeroplane.

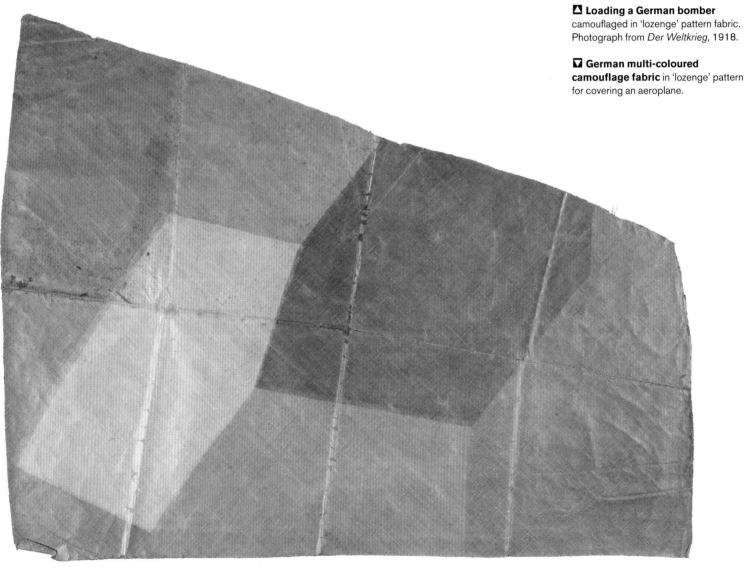

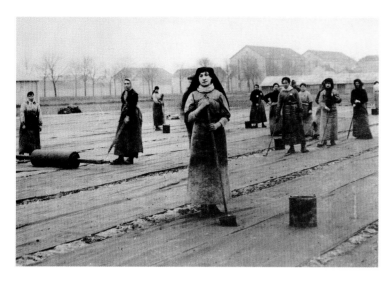

◩ **French peasants paint burlap** at an American camouflage factory on the Western Front.

▶ *A German Gunner's Shelter*, oil painting by William Orpen, 1917. A highly fashionable portrait painter before the war, Orpen was one of the first official war artists appointed by the British government. Shocked by what he witnessed at the Somme, he refused to make any profit from the pictures he completed during the war.

The Germans had been quicker off the mark than either the British or the French, Solomon argued, because they better understood the power of aerial reconnaissance. 'During the first days of the war,' he wrote, 'accounts were given of the part played by German airmen in marking the range of tactical positions for the benefit of her artillery.... Her aerial photography was at that time of a high order. Not until we captured a German aeroplane, and developed the plates found on it, did we know what the camera was capable of in this direction.'

This early mastery of aerial photography meant the Germans began their experiments in camouflage by studying photographs of the area to be protected. They then created accurate models allowing them to test the perfect camouflage solutions.

Understanding that normal buildings cast tell-tale shadows, the Germans created very gently sloping structures the size of several fields to cover up aircraft hangars. While the British might hide one soldiers' hut with netting, the Germans would take ten huts and spread gradually sloping covering material across them all to fit the contours of a farmer's field. While the British might erect a painted vertical screen to hide a road, the Germans would cover it over. It was the immensity and subtlety of these camouflage shelters that impressed Solomon. He also believed that the camouflaging of tens of thousands of German troops assembling behind the enemy frontline seriously misled Allied strategists.

To be fair to the British, their 1918 booklet, *The Principles and Practice of Camouflage*, does advocate the camouflaging of entire fields to cover batteries of guns, but Solomon contended that this large-scale approach came too late in the war and that the Germans were using it from 1914 onwards to disguise all their troop concentrations and movements. It was a stark lesson that Solomon hoped the British would learn from.

The United States did not enter the First World War until 1917, but quickly absorbed the camouflage lessons learned by its allies. Barry Faulkner, cousin to Abbott Thayer, the great natural historian and painter of camouflage in animals (see pages 20–23), established the New York Camouflage Society in a Greenwich Village studio. He then volunteered his services, along with several artists, to start a US camouflage unit as Company A of the US 40th Engineers, eventually setting up a camouflage workshop near Dijon in France.

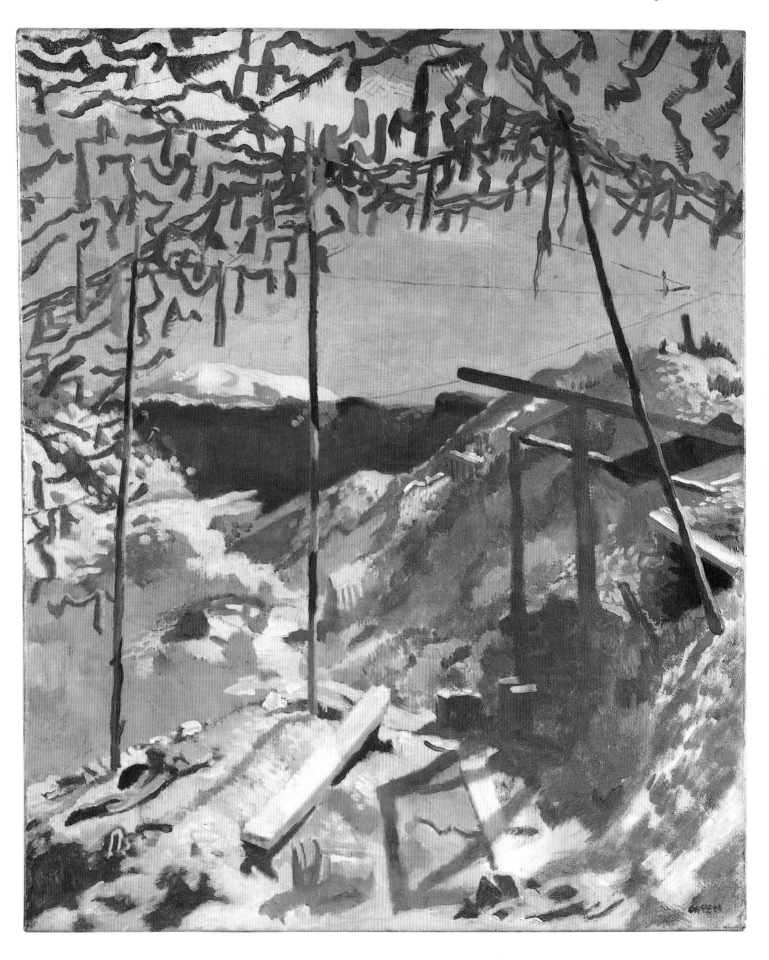

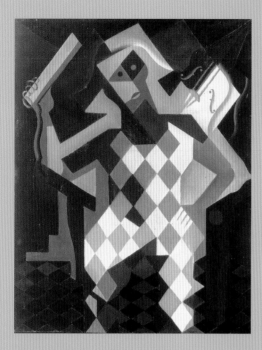

⬓ **The Harlequin**, oil painting by Juan Gris, 1918. This clown figure in multi-coloured lozenge-patterned costume was a favourite theme for Cubist artists, including Pablo Picasso, who even suggested it as a possible uniform for soldiers in the First World War.

▶ **Pages from a sketchbook by André Mare**. Working as a *camoufleur* on the Western Front, Mare was also an artist who produced his own modernist visions of the war. He included a self-portrait in uniform among his frontline studies (bottom left).

Cubism and Camouflage

When Pablo Picasso saw a camouflaged cannon in a Paris street during the First World War, he exclaimed 'C'est nous qui avons fait ça!' 'It is we who created that!' But how true is that? Did Cubism and modern art really inspire the disruptive patterns of military camouflage in the First World War?

Our source for this quote is the American author Gertrude Stein, who lived in Paris during the war and was close friends with Picasso and other avant-garde artists. Stein reported that Picasso was spellbound when he saw the camouflaged gun and she agreed with his conclusion, saying 'From Cézanne through him they had come to that.'

Stein may have recognized obvious parallels between the dislocated forms of Cubist art and the disruptive patterns of military camouflage, but that didn't necessarily mean that one directly influenced the other. Picasso himself was very little interested in the war and had little to do with it. Fellow originator of Cubism Georges Braque became an infantry officer and was almost killed in 1915 by a shrapnel wound to his head – he was still in hospital nine months later. When eventually discharged from the army, he was awarded the Légion d'Honneur and Croix de Guerre. Long after the war, Braque claimed some affinity with camouflage: '"Cubism and camouflage," I once said to someone. He answered that it was all coincidence. "No, no," I said, "it is you who are wrong. Before Cubism we had Impressionism, and the Army used pale blue uniforms, horizon blue, atmospheric camouflage."'

Roland Penrose, artist and *camoufleur* in the Second World War (see pages 92–96), reported a conversation between Picasso and the poet Jean Cocteau about military camouflage later in the war. 'If they want to make an army invisible at a distance,' said Picasso, 'they have only to dress their men as harlequins.' Penrose understood immediately what Picasso meant by this seemingly ridiculous idea. 'Harlequin, Cubism and military camouflage had joined hands,' Penrose concluded. 'The point they had in common was the disruption of their exterior form in a desire to change their too easily recognized identity.'

But although neither Picasso nor Braque played any direct part in the painting of military schemes, if we look beyond the most famous names of the period, we do see a close involvement between avant-garde artists and military camouflage. Cubist painter Jacques Villon, brother of sculptor Raymond Duchamp-Villon and Marcel Duchamp, served in the camouflage section of the French army. Before the war, Jacques and Raymond had been key figures in bringing together avant-garde artists and critics such as Francis Picabia, Robert Delaunay, and Fernand Léger. They exhibited together under the name 'Section d'Or' and in 1913 the two brothers showed their work at the influential Armory Show in New York.

Chief French *camoufleur* Lucien-Victor Guirand de Scévola made a point of employing artists associated with Cubism to paint artillery. This was despite patriotic French propaganda decrying modern, non-figurative art as '*l'art Boche*'. 'In order to deform totally the aspect of the object,' he later wrote, 'I had to employ the means that Cubists used to represent it.'

André Mare was involved with the Duchamp-Villon circle through his work on the Maison Cubiste, an exhibit at the Paris Salon des Beaux-Arts of 1912 consisting of a series of rooms painted in primary colours with modernist decoration and objects. Mare had begun his career as an artist but turned to avant-garde interior design from 1905 onwards. He later established a design company with Louis Sue that pioneered Art Deco style in France.

During the war, Mare was a senior figure in the French camouflage corps and a much-valued advisor to British *camoufleurs*. He was clearly very aware of Cubist ideas and made exquisite sketches of his wartime work that show a direct link between the art movement and military camouflage. These culminate in a double-page watercolour sketch in his notebook of 1917 showing a camouflaged 28cm gun. It is a brilliant piece of Cubist-style art combined with an accurate rendering of an artillery camouflage scheme.

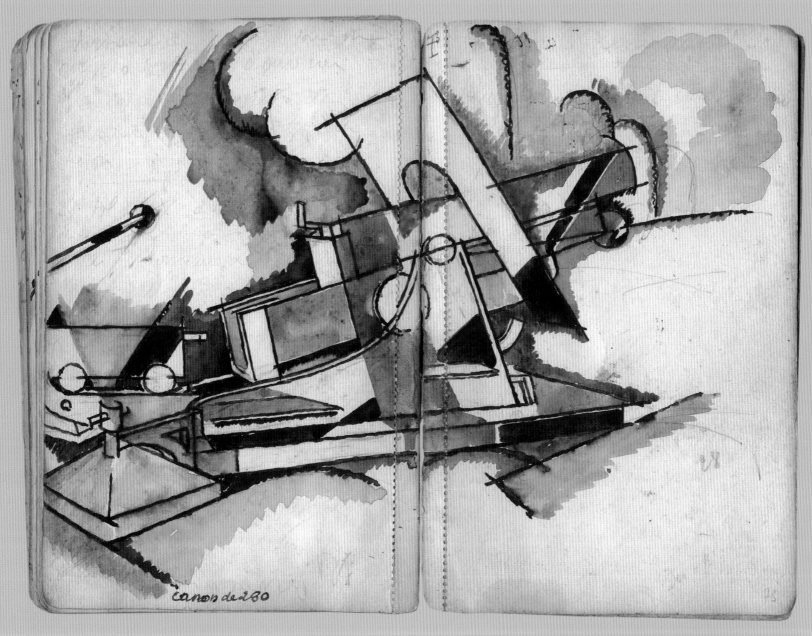

Canon de 280

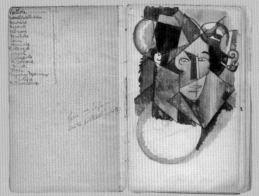

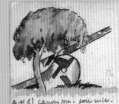

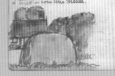

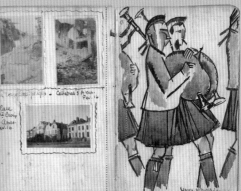

Razzle-Dazzle Ships

The most famous camouflage in the First World War was 'Dazzle', the boldly modernist and highly decorative disruptive pattern designs that were applied to British ships. Dazzle was the brain-child of Lieutenant-Commander Norman Wilkinson, who had been a traditional marine artist before the war. He later explained the concept behind it in a speech given in 1919:

'The primary object of this scheme,' said Wilkinson, 'was not so much to cause the enemy to miss his shot when actually in firing position, but to mislead him, when the ship was first sighted, as to the correct position to take up.' Dazzle was a 'method to produce an effect by paint in such a way that all accepted forms of a ship are broken up by masses of strongly contrasted colour, consequently making it a matter of difficulty for a submarine to decide on the exact course of the vessel to be attacked.'

Its main aim was to upset the targeting of German U-boat commanders and there is some evidence that it worked. 'It was not until she was within half a mile,' said one U-boat captain, 'that I could make out she was one ship steering a course at right angles, crossing from starboard to port. The dark painted stripes on her after part made her stern appear her bow, and a broad cut of green paint amidships looks like a patch of water. The weather was bright and visibility good; this was the best camouflage I have ever seen.'

◩ ◪ **Plans and drawings for Dazzle camouflage** on the H.M.S. *King Alfred*. These are signed by Norman Wilkinson, the Lieutenant-Commander who pioneered the development of Dazzle camouflage patterns for British naval and merchant ships during the First World War.

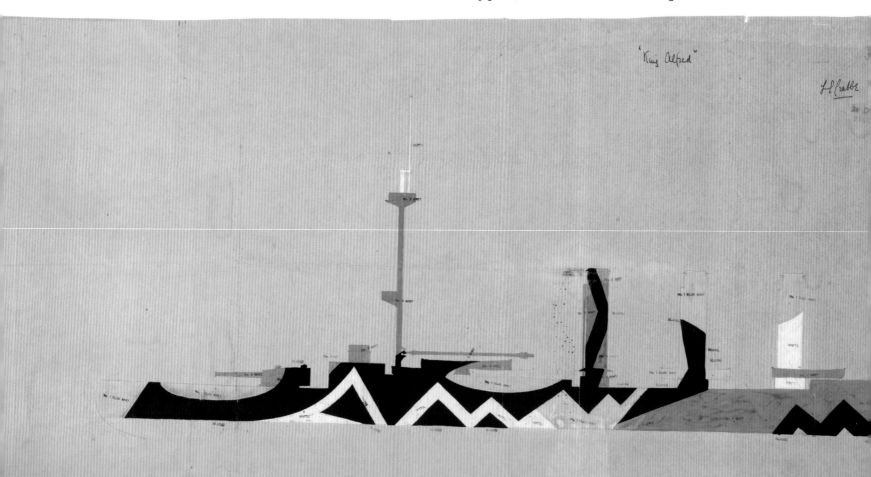

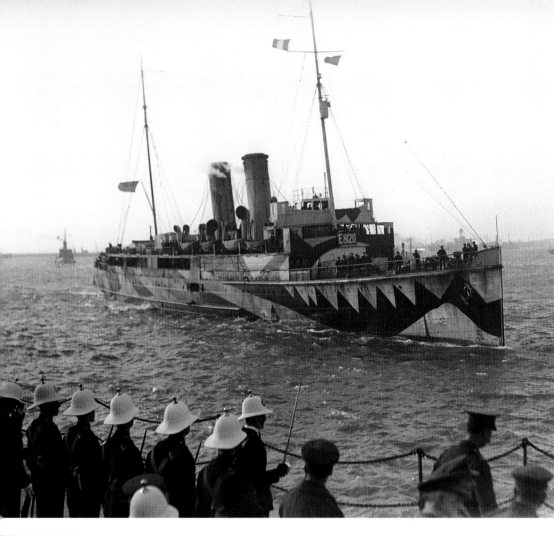

◀ **A ship bearing Dazzle camouflage** brings British Commander-in-Chief Sir Douglas Haig into port in 1919.

OVERLEAF Model ships painted in a variety of Dazzle camouflage patterns to designs by Lieutenant-Commander Norman Wilkinson. Once decorated, each model – measuring some 10 inches (25 centimetres) in length – would be viewed at a distance through a periscope in the studio to see if the pattern successfully deceived the eye.

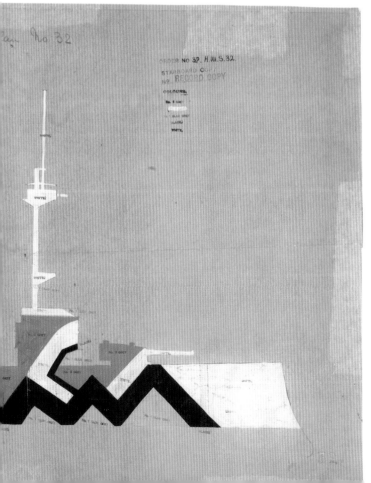

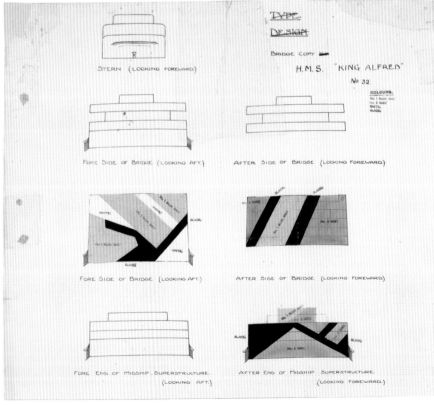

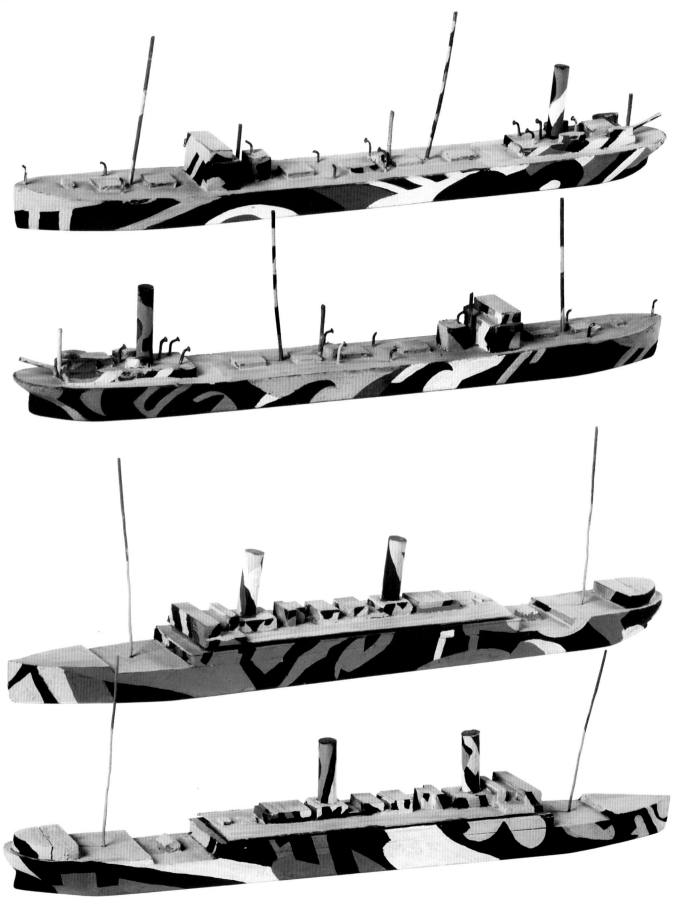

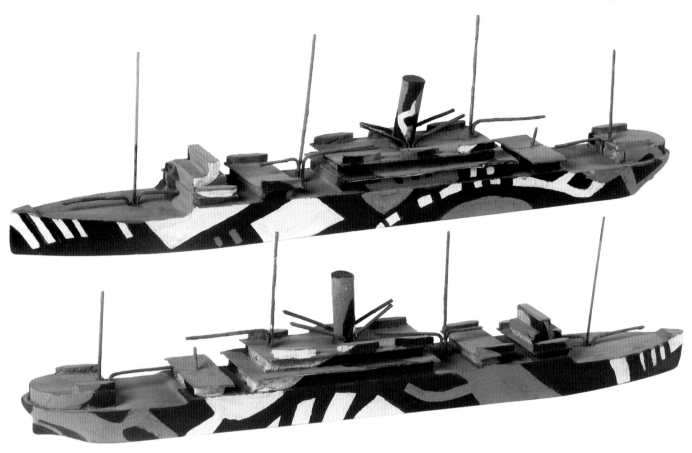

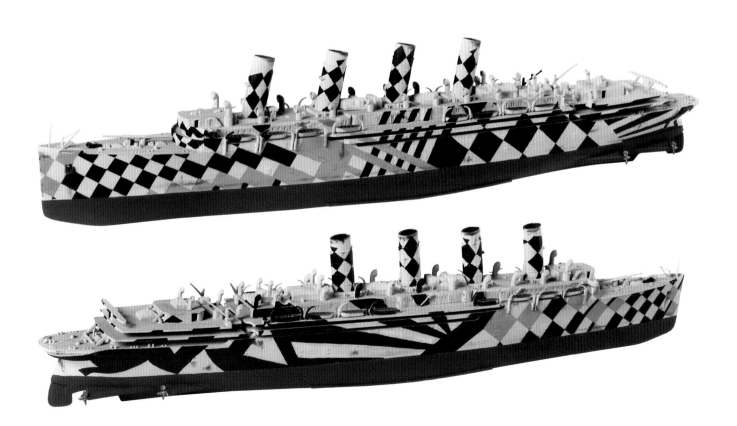

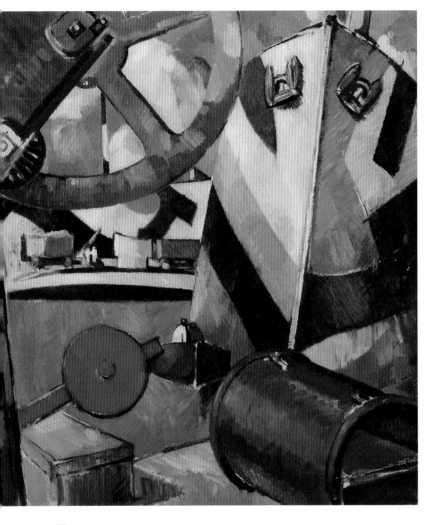

⬈ Dockyard, Portsmouth, oil painting by John Duncan Fergusson, 1918, showing a Dazzle-painted ship in the dock. Fergusson lived in France from 1905 and was strongly influenced by European avant-garde artists such as the Fauves.

⬊ Herculaneum Dock, ink and watercolour by L. Campbell Taylor, 1919. A brilliant rendition of a Dazzle-painted transport ship moored in Liverpool during the First World War.

Trial schemes must have been a success as by October 1917, the British Admiralty decided to paint all its merchant ships in Dazzle designs. Patterns were first tested on wooden models viewed through a periscope in a studio. Many of the designs were painted by women artists working in the Royal Academy of Arts in London. If deemed successful, the designs would then be presented to a foreman who had the task of scaling them up for the real thing.

'The colours mostly in use,' said Wilkinson, 'were black, white, blue and green, either in their primary condition, or mixed to various tones. When making a design for a vessel, vertical lines were largely avoided. Sloping lines, curves and stripes are by far the best and give the greater distortion.'

They also gave the ships a jazzy modern look. As with army camouflage sections, the work of creating Dazzle ships attracted many artists. The most famous of these was Edward Wadsworth. He was serving as a naval intelligence officer in the Mediterranean when he was recruited by Wilkinson, and he leapt at the opportunity. He oversaw Dazzle painting at Bristol and Liverpool docks and then went on to produce a series of woodcuts and paintings capturing the strange spectacle of Dazzle ships.

During the war Wilkinson travelled to the United States to give advice on Dazzle painting to the US naval authorities, but the Americans had already been talking to George de Forest Brush, a painter colleague of Abbott Thayer, and they developed Dazzle schemes of their own. By the end of the war, 1,256 American merchant ships were camouflaged and it was claimed that less than one per cent of them fell victim to German torpedoes.

The British Admiralty set up a committee to research the true worth of Dazzle painting and in September 1918 it reported there was no evidence to prove that the enemy had been confused by the painted schemes. The committee did concede, however, that 'in view of the undoubted increase in confidence and morale of Officers and Crews of the Merchant Marine resulting from this painting...it may be found advisable to continue the system though probably not under the present wholesale conditions.'

Camouflage as a lucky military charm – more about psychology than practicality – was to be a recurring theme throughout its use in war.

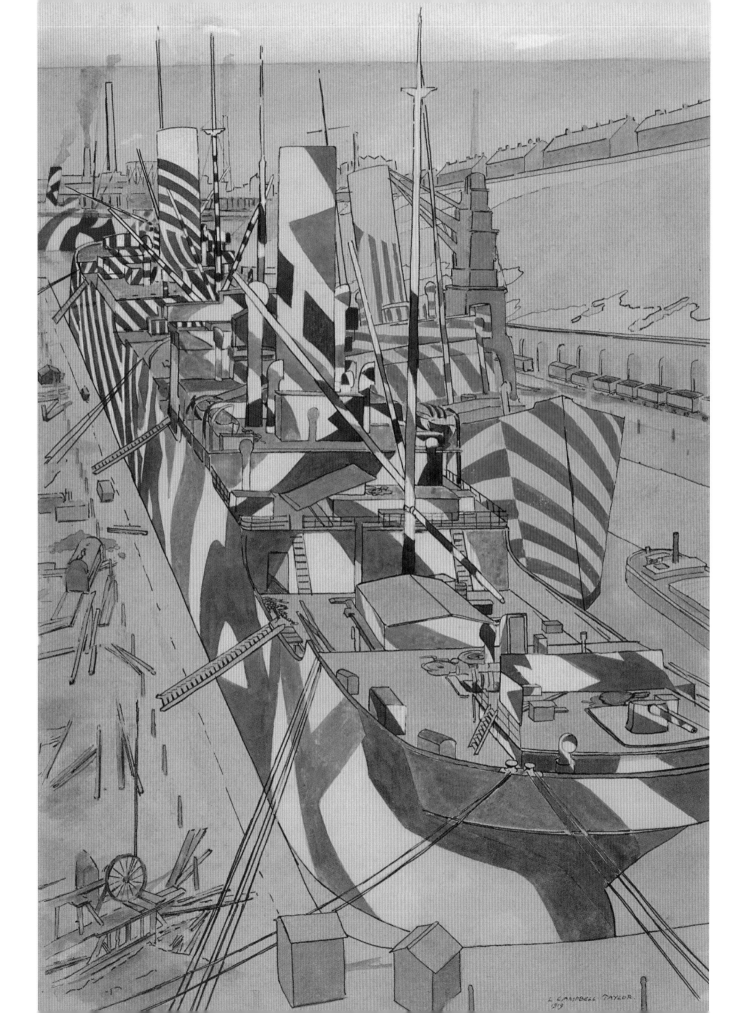

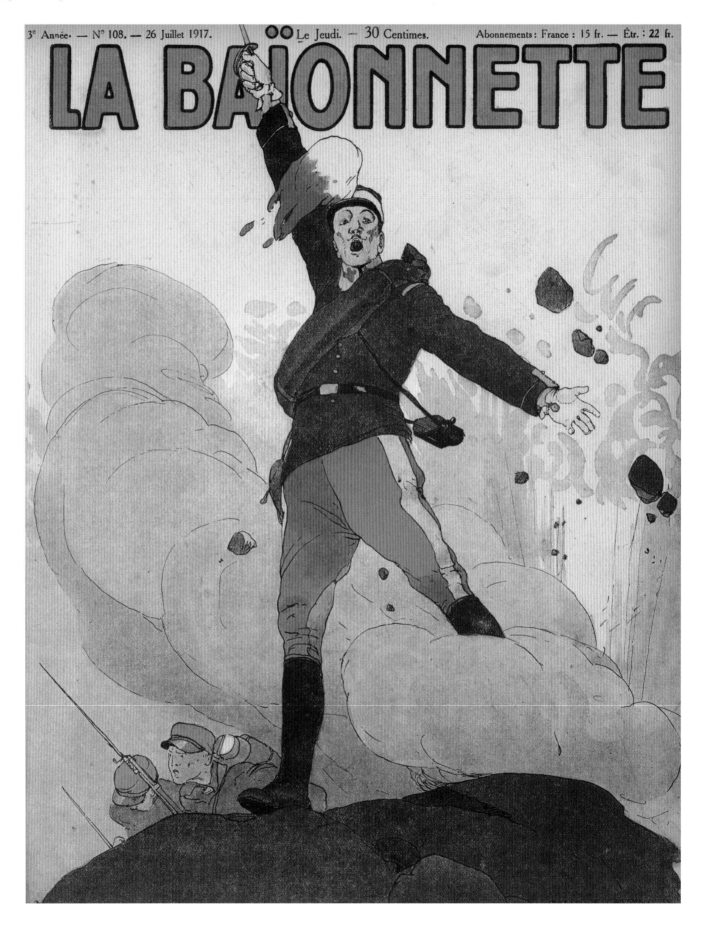

3e Année. — N° 108. — 26 Juillet 1917.　○○ Le Jeudi. — 30 Centimes.　Abonnements : France : 15 fr. — Étr. : 22 fr.

LA BAÏONNETTE

Personal Camouflage

Although disruptive pattern camouflage was used on artillery, tanks, aircraft and ships, the idea of applying it to individual soldiers' clothing was not widely adopted in the First World War. Throughout the entire conflict, most armies wore single colour combat uniforms. The British wore khaki and the Germans field grey. There were a few notable exceptions. The French army went to war in dark blue tunics and red trousers. This made their soldiers easy targets, and prompted a change to 'horizon blue' soon after the war began. This change was often not reflected in illustrations of soldiers in the popular press, however, for the French public still preferred to see their soldiers depicted in more heroic-seeming bright red trousers.

In France, pioneering experiments were conducted by Eugène Corbin, working at the Magasins Réunis department store in Nancy.

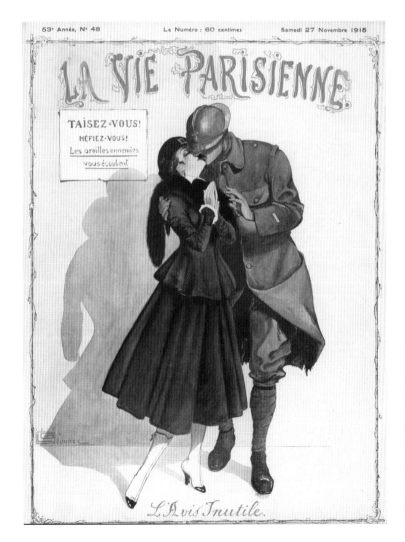

◀◀ **A French Lieutenant strikes a heroic pose** to encourage his men. Magazine cover by De Gastyne for *La Baïonnette*, July 1917. Despite most French soldiers wearing 'horizon blue' by this time, many popular illustrations continued to show them in bright red trousers.

◀ **'Horizon blue' combat uniform**, as worn by the soldier in this illustration, was rather more sensible. Magazine cover by G. Leonnec for *La Vie Parisienne*, November 1915.

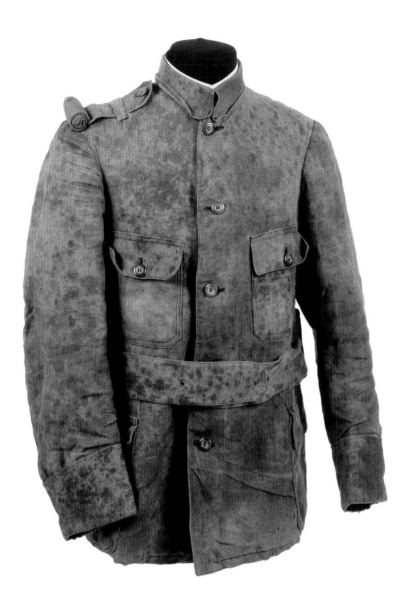

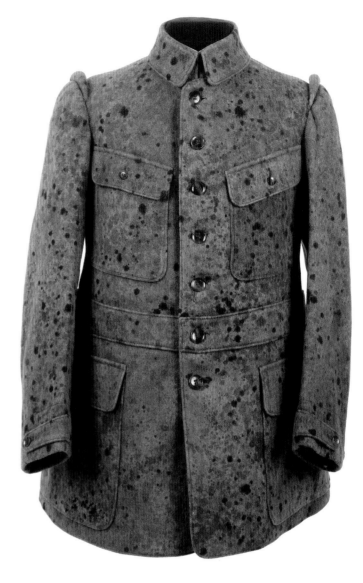

◤▷ **Camouflaged tunics and overalls designed by Eugène Corbin**, a French *camoufleur* working at the Magasins Réunis department store in Nancy. He painted these experimental camouflage outfits around 1916. The designs did not go into production.

Around 1916, Corbin produced a camouflaged uniform, including a waistcoat, in a scheme of green and blue spattered paint. It was not so much disruptive pattern as pointillist. It did not go into mass production. Even had the French military authorities wanted to adopt it, the technology to mass produce such a textile did not exist in 1916.

In the British Army, sharpshooters were equipped with sniping suits that consisted of loose hooded robes that reached to below the knee. These sniper robes were individually hand-painted. One of several surviving examples (overleaf) indicates their colour range. Made of canvas, it is basically khaki drab in colour with dark earth and dark green paint daubed over it to create a disruptive pattern. Another type of sniper outfit made with trousers appeared in 1916 and was called a 'crawling suit'.

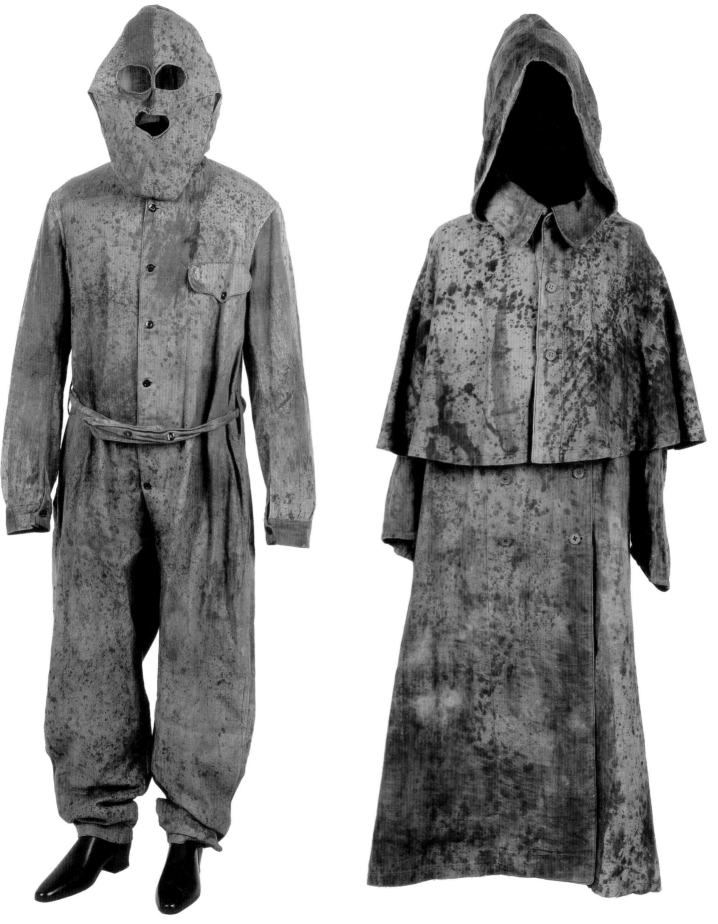

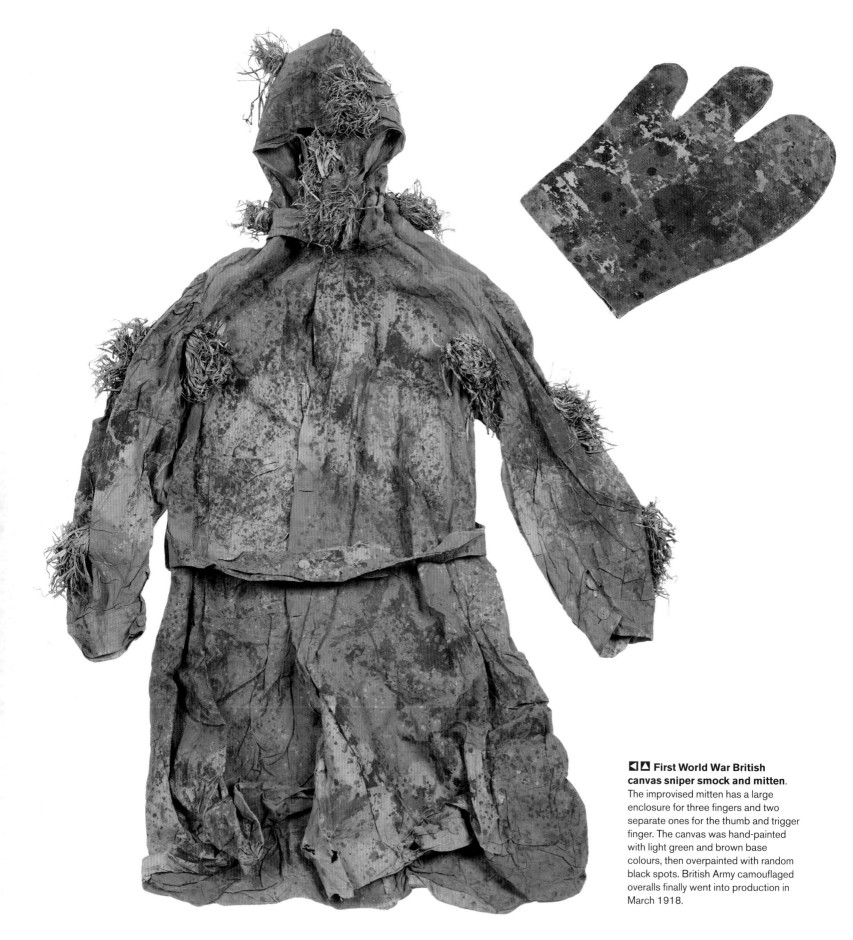

◀◥ **First World War British canvas sniper smock and mitten**. The improvised mitten has a large enclosure for three fingers and two separate ones for the thumb and trigger finger. The canvas was hand-painted with light green and brown base colours, then overpainted with random black spots. British Army camouflaged overalls finally went into production in March 1918.

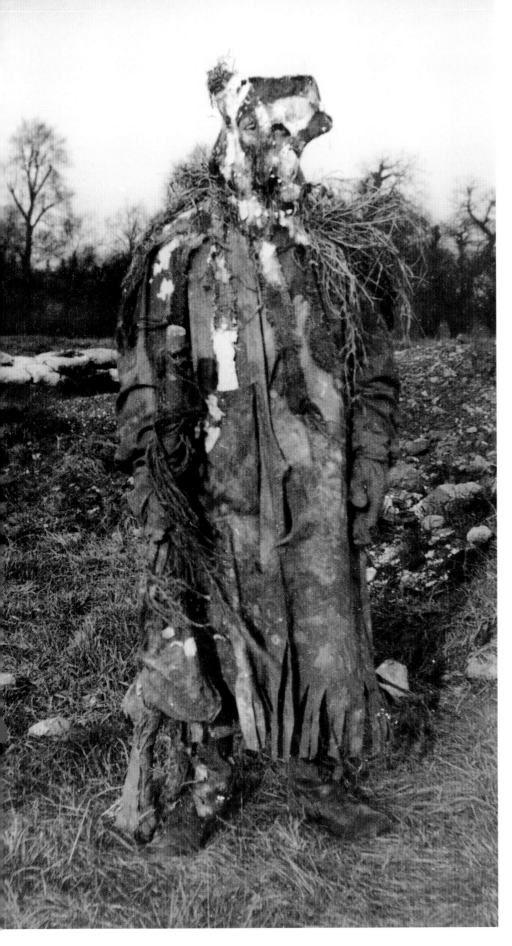

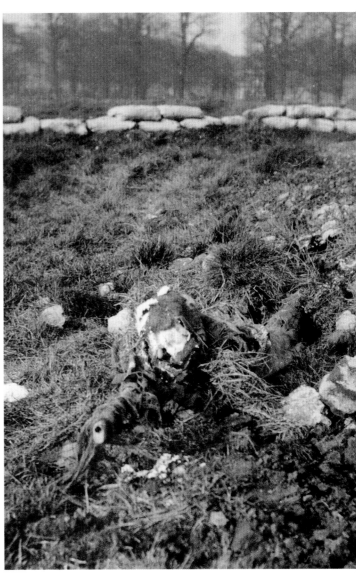

◄ **First World War British sniper** in camouflage smock with attached foliage.

▼ **British sniper** concealed on the ground.

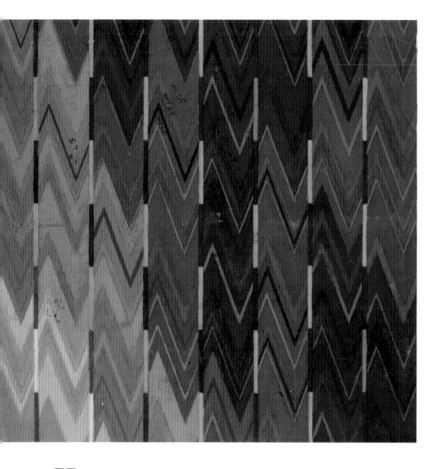

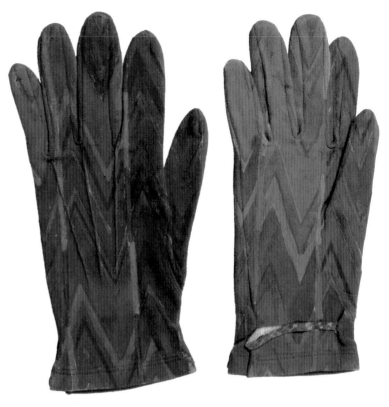

◣◥ **Experimental camouflage pattern** applied to sniper gloves and sniper suit material, designed by Percyval Tudor-Hart, 1917. Hand-painted in oil on cotton, the striking camouflage outfit was presented to the British War Office, who considered it no better than their current sniper suits. The pattern was tested for use on tanks and even suggested as camouflage for ships, but was finally ruled out.

By March 1918, two further forms of camouflaged overall were in production in Britain: a boiler suit type with a detachable hood of scrim (loosely woven fabric to which foliage can be attached), rifle cover and gloves; and a more modern-looking, so-called Symien sniper suit consisting entirely of loose-fitting scrim with a hood attached, separate leggings, rifle cover and gloves. White snow suits were also produced, as was a dark brown night-time overall. These were an early indication of what camouflage clothing could achieve, but as soon as the war ended, such innovation ceased and it would be over a decade before camouflage clothing appeared again in the British Army.

In the German army, soldiers painted their new-style steel helmet – the *Stahlhelm* – with brightly coloured disruptive patterns. Painted with browns, greens, yellows and reds, these camouflaged helmets were worn most famously by trench-assaulting 'stormtroopers' from 1917 onwards. The idea never spread to their uniforms and it would take another war before disruptive pattern became more widely used.

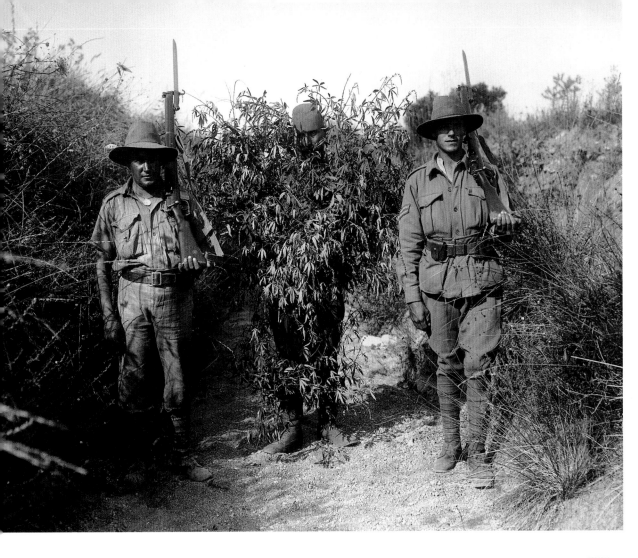

▲ **Turkish sniper** captured at Gallipoli and escorted by Australian soldiers.

▶ **German *Stahlhelm*** painted in disruptive camouflage pattern. This was the only item of camouflaged combat uniform worn by the German army and was used by trench-assaulting 'stormtroopers' from 1917 onwards.

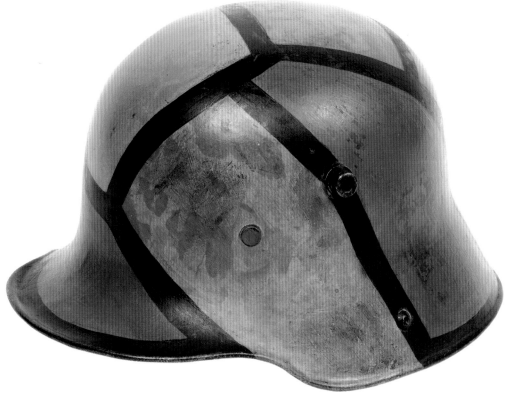

◥ ***Ju-Jitsu***, oil painting by David Bomberg, *c.* 1913. Dazzle-style patterns and the psychology of perception were explored by the British artist before their use in the First World War. Bomberg served in the British Army from 1915 to 1919.

▷ **A Dazzle-inspired dress** worn by photographer Yvonne Gregory in a 1919 portrait by her husband Bertram Park.

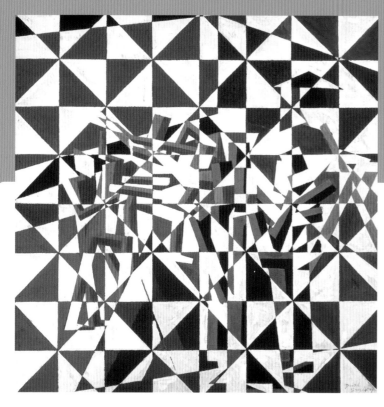

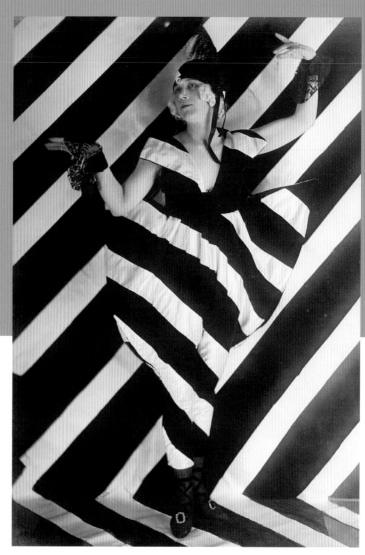

The Dazzle Ball

Just four months after the Armistice brought an end to the fighting in the First World War, there was anxiety about whether it was appropriate to hold large parties in London before a formal peace treaty had been signed. 'Will there be a season or won't there?' enquired *The Illustrated London News* in March 1919. 'That is the question. It would certainly seem that there can be no certainty until international and industrial peace is secure.'

But people were yearning for normality and the Chelsea Arts Club took the plunge. It resumed its famous themed balls in London and the first one, early in 1919, took the inspiration of wartime

camouflage. It was held in the ballroom of the Royal Albert Hall on the evening of 12 March. *The Times* correspondent was there and was struck by the strange Dazzle costumes signifying a new age of freer expression.

'Here, it seemed,' he wrote, 'was a token, unmistakeable if bizarre, of some of the things which the dark years have achieved, of the breaking of bonds, of the setting free of the spirits which dwell within the forms of things…

'To the strains of the Jazz band these amazing revellers, vanishing and reappearing, seemed to set at naught the world of the past and all the

portentousness of it. They hailed a new world, swifter, gayer, more adventurous.'

The Times correspondent credited the invention of Dazzle to Lieutenant-Commander Norman Wilkinson and his Royal Navy colleagues, and described how their schemes were adapted to costumes. 'The very fact,' he observed, 'that this disruptive colouration broke up the usual lines of form gave to many of the costumes a grace and charm as delightful as they were unexpected…. Even the freakish creations held the suggestion of a new kind of wonder, the 'camouflage' of men and women…

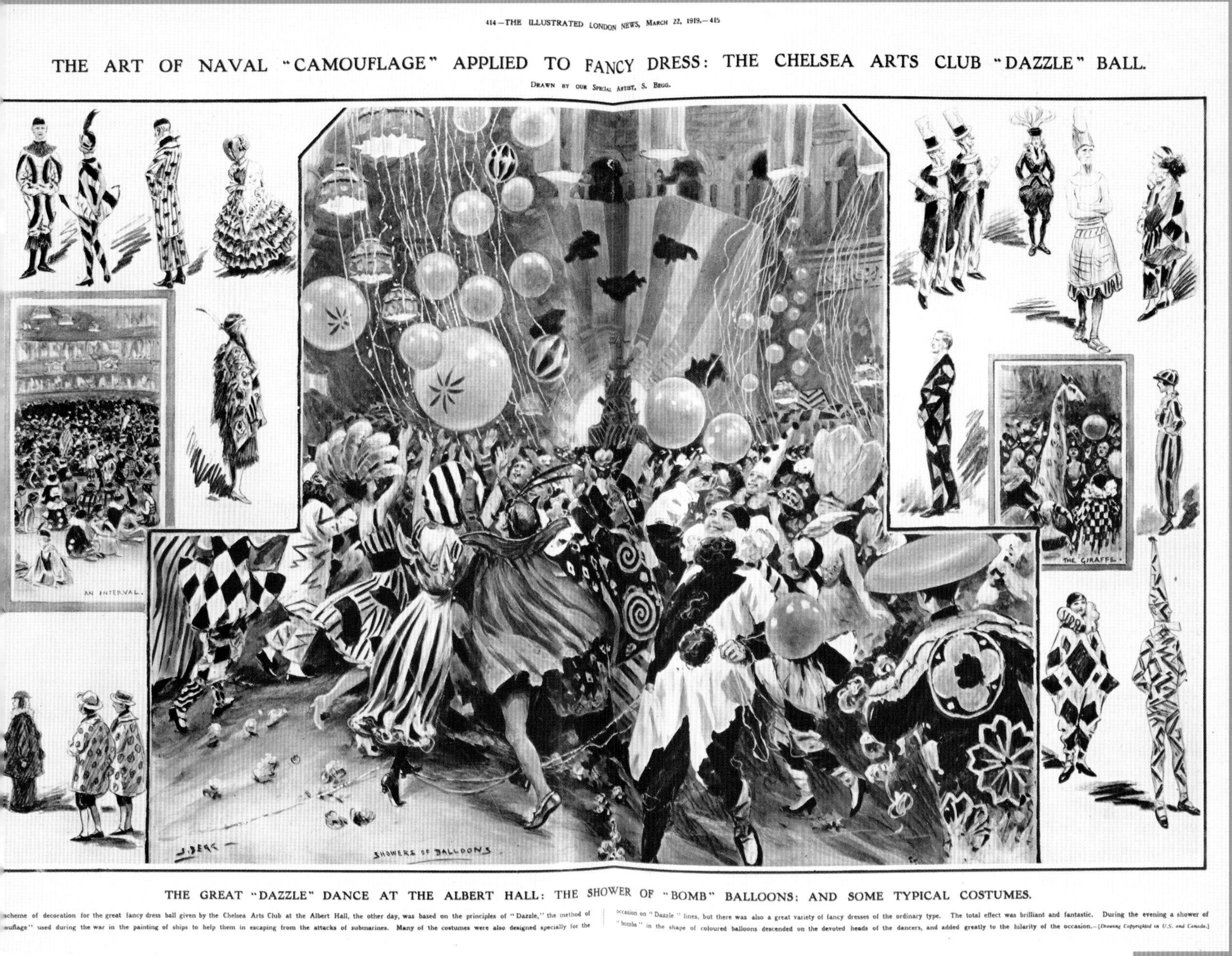

414—THE ILLUSTRATED LONDON NEWS, MARCH 22, 1919.—415

THE ART OF NAVAL "CAMOUFLAGE" APPLIED TO FANCY DRESS: THE CHELSEA ARTS CLUB "DAZZLE" BALL.

DRAWN BY OUR SPECIAL ARTIST, S. BEGG.

THE GREAT "DAZZLE" DANCE AT THE ALBERT HALL: THE SHOWER OF "BOMB" BALLOONS: AND SOME TYPICAL COSTUMES.

scheme of decoration for the great fancy dress ball given by the Chelsea Arts Club at the Albert Hall, the other day, was based on the principles of "Dazzle," the method of ouflage" used during the war in the painting of ships to help them in escaping from the attacks of submarines. Many of the costumes were also designed specially for the occasion on "Dazzle" lines, but there was also a great variety of fancy dresses of the ordinary type. The total effect was brilliant and fantastic. During the evening a shower of "bombs" in the shape of coloured balloons descended on the devoted heads of the dancers, and added greatly to the hilarity of the occasion.—[Drawing Copyrighted in U.S. and Canada.]

'One might be forgiven for not expecting wholly to relish the spectacle of Cubist birds, Futurist animals, submarines, Messrs Dilly and Dally, impish pierettes, Geisha girls, demons, fairies, staff officers, and officers of the Grand Fleet jostling one another under multi-coloured searchlights that flashed and scintillated. But one did relish it. Enjoyment was of the spirit of the hour.'

The Illustrated London News devoted a picture spread to the Dazzle Ball in an effort to capture its brilliance. Its artist sketched some of the camouflage-inspired costumes, and also noted that other costumes were worn, including harlequin clowns – a favourite theme of Cubist artists.

This extraordinary spectacle makes clear the extent to which wartime camouflage had fired the public imagination. It is also the very first significant demonstration of camouflage being taken up by popular culture – a trend otherwise still several decades in the future.

▲ The Dazzle Ball at the Royal Albert Hall in March 1919, as depicted in the *The Illustrated London News*. Alongside the Dazzle costumes inspired by Norman Wilkinson's naval designs, there are also harlequin costumes, a favourite theme of Cubist painters at the time.

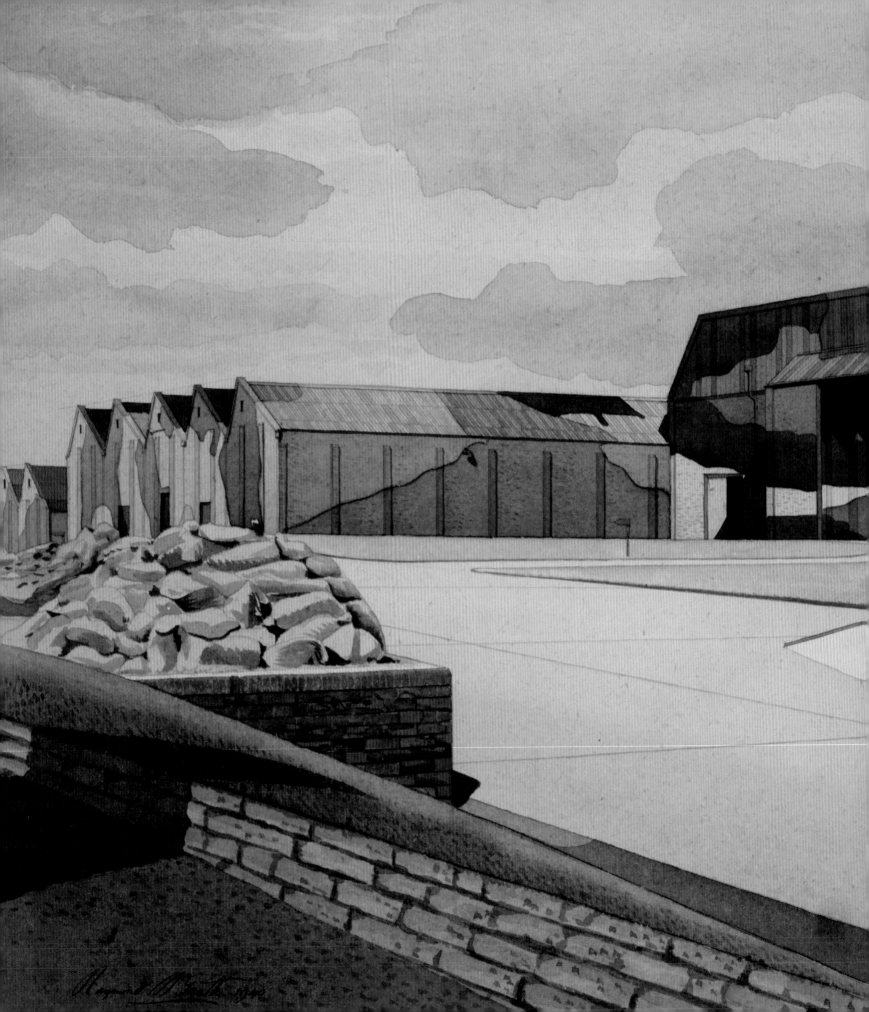

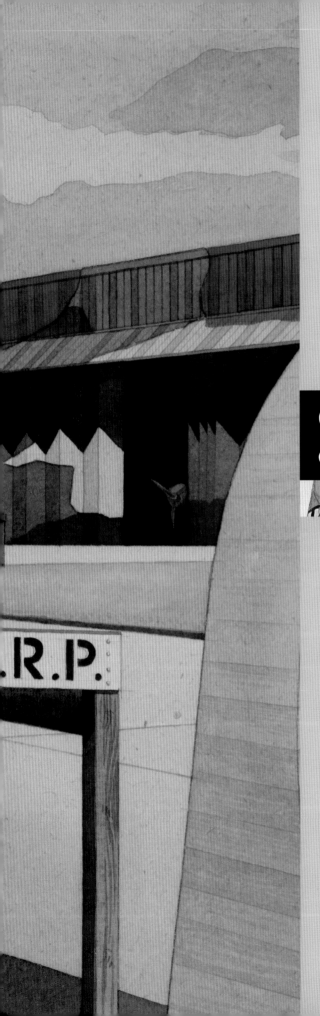

Camouflaging a Nation
Camouflage in the Second World War

The Second World War saw camouflage pursued on an altogether greater scale. Not only military bases and equipment were screened and disguised, but factories, airfields and railways. In a situation of total warfare, thousands of civilians participated in this monumental task. Disruptive pattern uniforms were also now issued to large numbers of individual soldiers.

Camouflaging a Nation
Camouflage in the Second World War

Previous page: *Hangars*,
watercolour by Raymond McGrath,
1940. A row of British aircraft hangars
painted with camouflage patterns.

⬇ **English Surrealist** Roland Penrose
turned his skills to teaching and
lecturing on camouflage during the
Second World War. But as the
disruptive pattern painted on his car
reveals, he did not lose the sense of
playful absurdity that typified the
Surrealist movement.

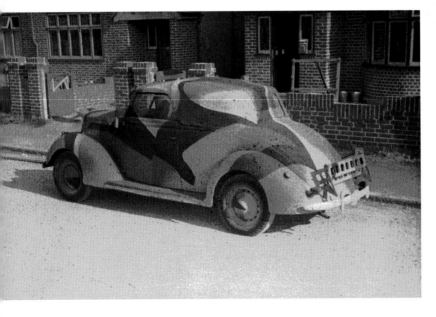

In 1936, English Surrealism burst onto the scene with an exhibition at the New Burlington Galleries in London. It was organized by Roland Penrose, a Surrealist painter and collector then in his mid-30s. His greatest coup was to get Salvador Dalí to turn up at the private view and give a lecture while wearing a diving suit and holding two white greyhounds on a leash. Four years later, Roland Penrose would be giving lectures to a completely different audience – the British Home Guard. But he was still a Surrealist at heart and included slides of his lover, Lee Miller, naked and covered only in camouflage cream and netting to keep his audience interested.

Surrealist Advice

Roland Penrose was an excellent communicator and wrote a booklet called the *Home Guard Manual of Camouflage*. It was a thorough analysis of the nature and application of camouflage. He devoted a chapter to camouflage in the natural world and then showed how these lessons could be applied by the Home Guard to the defence of their country. As in the First World War, the great challenge was to defy enemy aerial photography in black and white.

'In order to obtain concealment,' instructed Penrose, 'it would appear at first sight that resemblance in colour is the most important factor. Actually, this is not the case. The fact is that a smooth surface reflects more light than a rough surface. In consequence, supposing we have a smooth board and rough piece of bath towel, both painted with exactly the same colour, the smooth board will inevitably look light in tone.'

Penrose explained it was more important to match the texture of the background than its colour. A coat of paint alone would not do the job. This was because aerial photography eliminated colour from its observations but accentuated differences in tone.

As an artist, Penrose understood the nature of colours and pigments and explained that green – the most obvious colour to use in any camouflage scheme – had a basic flaw in that it usually contained too much blue in its mixture.

'There is very little blue-green in nature,' he said, 'also, when a green paint contains too much blue there is every probability that in time the yellow in it will fade and the resulting colour appear even more blue...owing to the persistence of the Prussian blue that is frequently used in green paint.'

The Home Guard had limited resources and so Penrose looked to cheap, easily available materials. He realized that many Home Guards were deployed as aircraft spotters and needed to camouflage their faces as they looked upwards. 'A mixture of soot and flour will make a good paste which sticks to the skin,' he

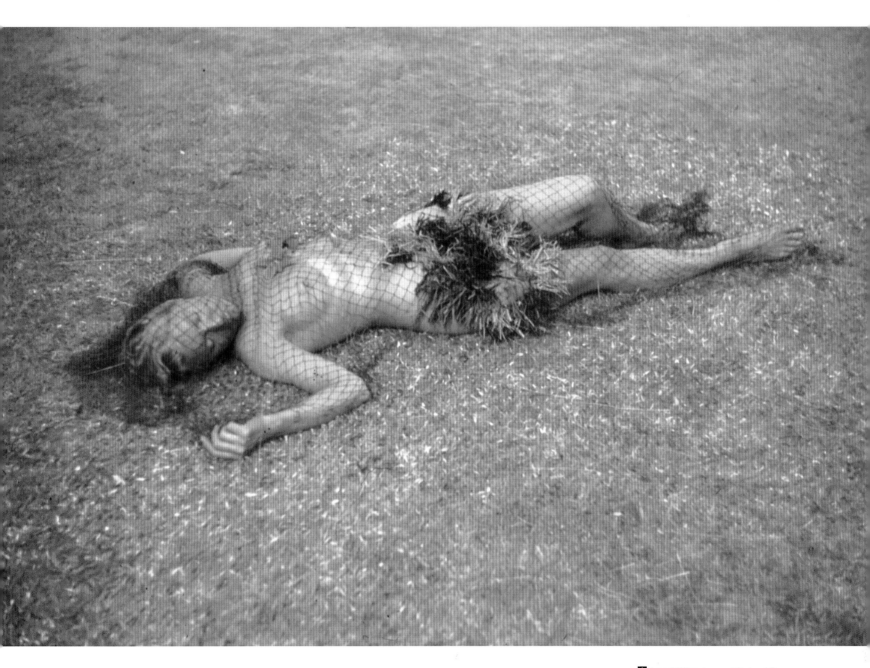

△ **Lee Miller**, lover of Roland Penrose, covered in camouflage cream and netting. Penrose used this photograph to enliven his lectures on camouflage to the British Home Guard.

recommended. 'By some who live in country districts cow-dung has been advocated, and for those who have the courage to use it, it can be highly recommended in spite of its unpleasantness, since it retains good colour and texture when dry.'

Net curtains were recommended as a good basic camouflage material for personal coverage, while insulating tape could be wound round the barrel of a rifle. He suggested ways of making sniper suits that included painting a boiler suit and then using a shrimp net to cover the head, or making a sniper suit out of hessian or sacking and then painting it with a disruptive pattern.

Penrose's excellent manual is just one of a whole library of camouflage instruction booklets produced in Britain during the Second World War. They demonstrate that the lessons of the First World War had been taken on board and that the British authorities now viewed camouflage as a very important element of both

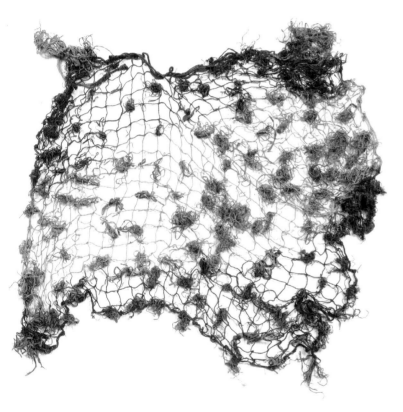

◤ **German camouflage netting**. This would be interwoven with local foliage and used for covering a soldier.

▶ **Japanese camouflage sniper shirt**. In the Second World War, the Japanese army wore no camouflage printed uniforms, but local foliage was used to disguise individual soldiers.

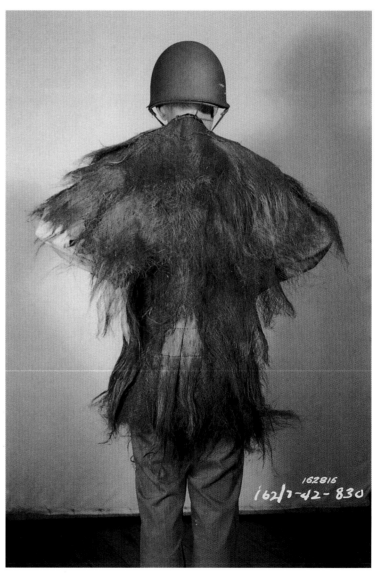

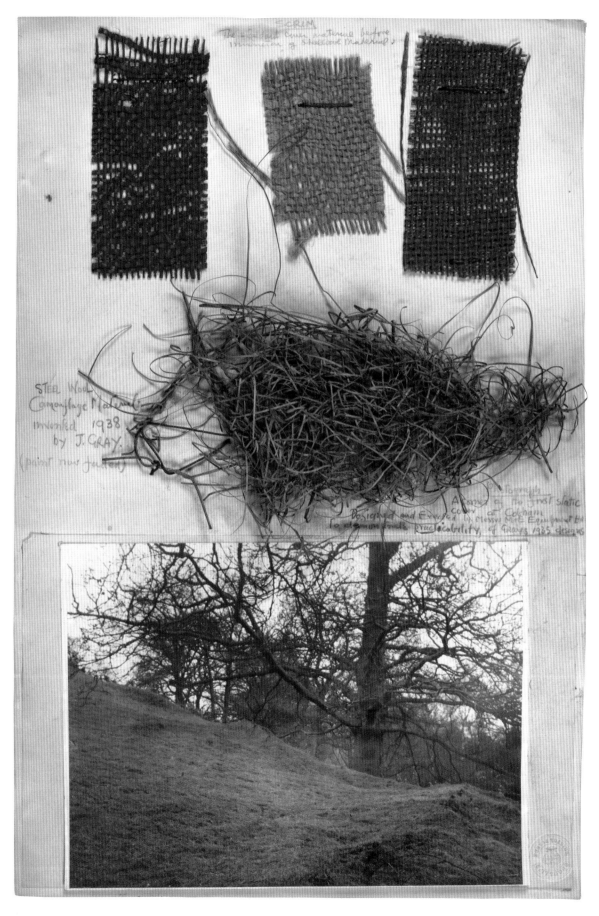

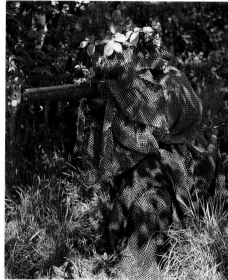

▲ **British sniper** in camouflage hood and shirt.

◄ **Steel wool garnish**, more durable than organic foliage, could also be attached to camouflage netting.

civil and military defence. It also showed that camouflage, by its very nature, attracted some leading visual and creative talents.

British military camouflage research was carried out at the Camouflage Development and Training Centre at Farnham Castle in Surrey, opened in 1940. Penrose was trained there, as was the celebrated magician Jasper Maskelyne, who went on to become a camouflage officer in North Africa. Maskelyne had been bored by the natural history talks: 'I think I may say, without particular vanity, that a lifetime of hiding things on the stage taught me more about the subject than rabbits and tigers will ever know.' Though sadly, vanity does seem to have got the better of Maskelyne, whose many grandiose claims for the military significance of the camouflage schemes devised by him and his 'Magic Gang' in North Africa are contested by recent research.

◗◗ **Studio photograph by Lee Miller** showing a man wearing camouflage cream and a garnished helmet. The aesthetic qualities of camouflage fascinated both Miller and Penrose.

◗ **Instructions to the British Home Guard** on how to maker a cheap and effective camouflage outfit.

▼ **Experiments in disruptive-pattern** camouflage clothing. This soldier wears a hand-painted sniper suit created by Roland Penrose. The photograph was taken by Lee Miller.

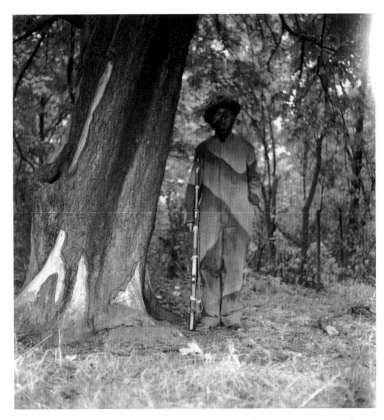

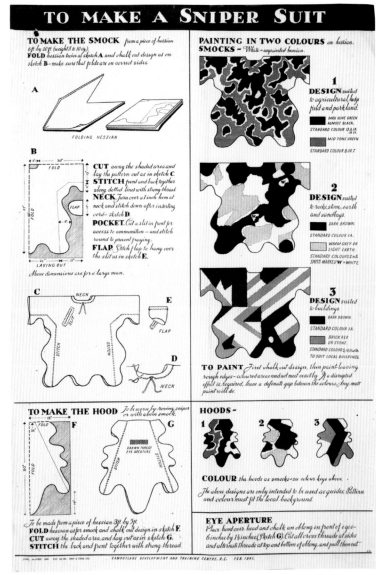

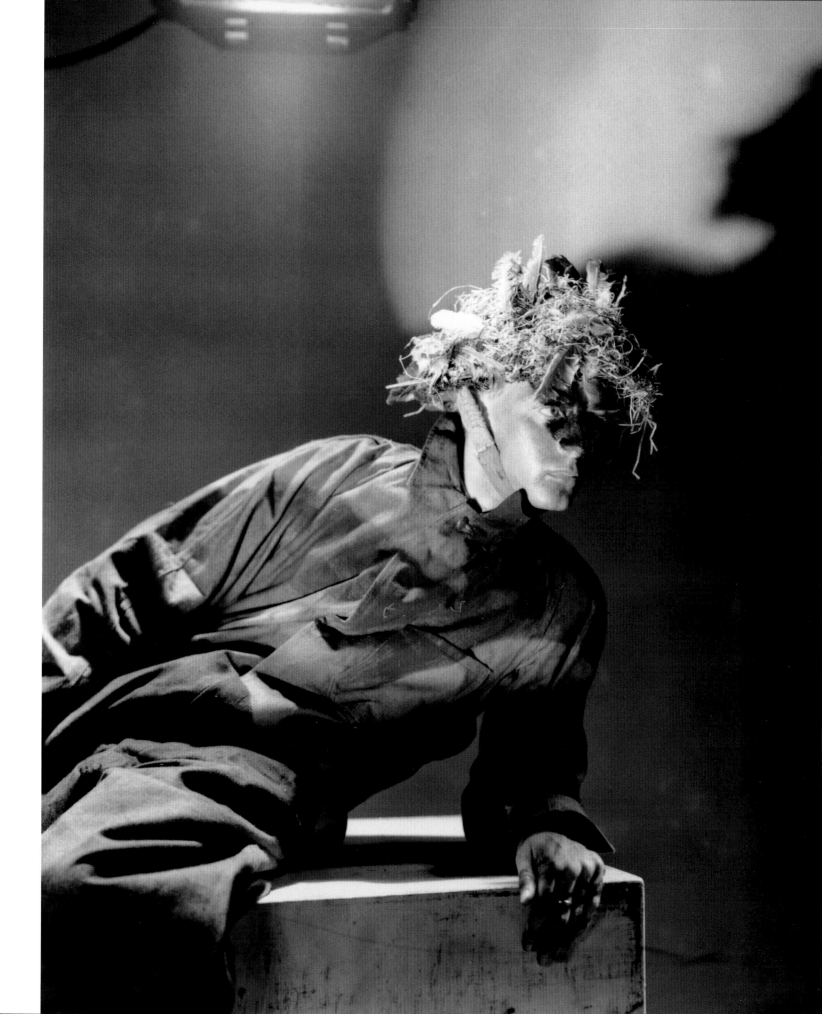

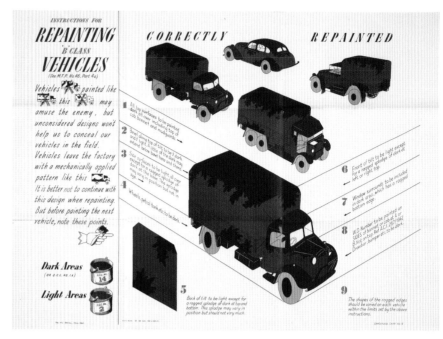

▶ **British wartime poster offering instructions for repainting vehicles** so that they presented less of a target to the enemy.

▼ **Poster explaining 'Personal Concealment'** to British Home Guard volunteers. This was less about colour and disruptive pattern and more about positioning and how to remain inconspicuous in open countryside.

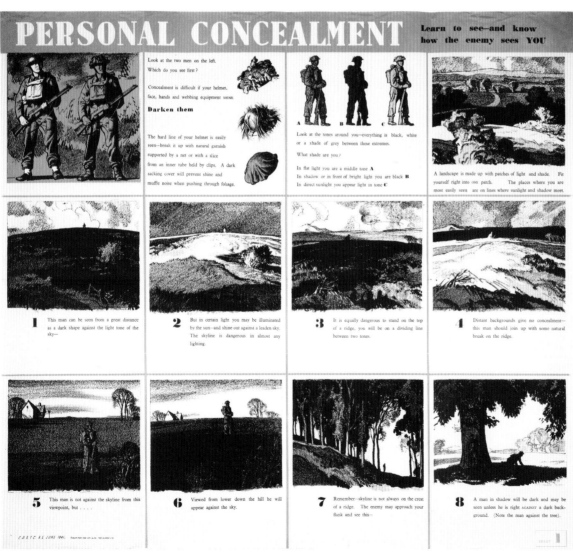

Poster explaining how to
conceal weapons and vehicles from
detection by aerial reconnaissance.
The high quality and inventiveness of
such official communications indicates
the importance the British authorities
placed upon camouflage during the
Second World War.

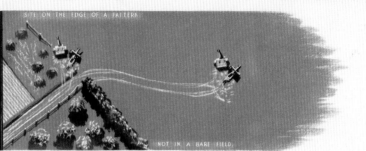
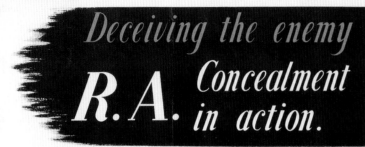

Deceiving the enemy
R.A. *Concealment in action.*

SITE ON THE EDGE OF A PATTERN

NOT IN A BARE FIELD.

USE OF ARTILLERY NETS AND LOCAL MATERIALS FOR TEMPORARY POSITIONS

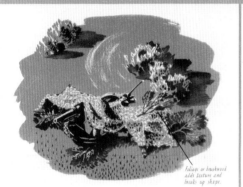
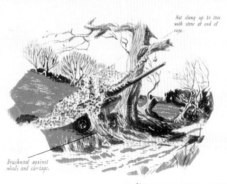
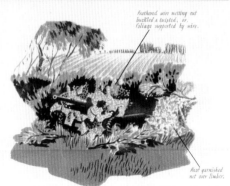

Net as a Drape { *Net draped over gun & limber to reduce shine.*

Linked to tree { *Net acts as a screen merging gun with winter tree.*

Screen of foliage { *A th gun shield merged into hedge with natural or artificial foliage.*

USE OF ARTILLERY NETS AND FRAMES TO COVER MESS AROUND DUG-IN POSITIONS

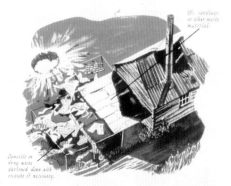
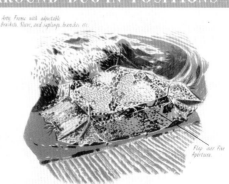

Linked to shed { *Patches to suggest broken ground and roof of a lean-to.*

Flat top cover { *Gun linked to hedge, local garnish added to cover.*

Mounded cover { *Mound extended from existing bank. Addition of local garnish.*

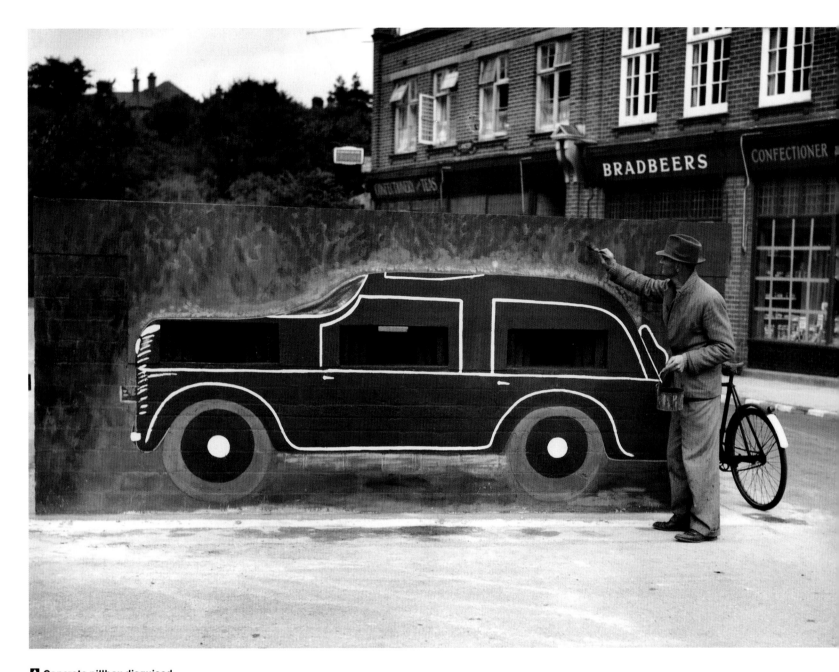

▲ **Concrete pillbox disguised as a car.** This is a crude attempt at camouflage that completely misunderstands how it works. It was partly to counter such naivety that the British authorities issued a wide range of camouflage instruction posters and booklets, and devoted resources to teaching camouflage skills to the Home Guard.

One colleague at Farnham was scathing. Maskelyne 'entertained us with his tricks in the evenings,' remembered Julian Trevelyan, 'and tried, rather unsuccessfully, to apply his techniques to the disguise of the concrete pill-boxes that were then appearing every-where overnight. He was at once innocent and urbane, and he ended up as an Entertainments officer in the Middle East.'

One of the natural history specialists who brought his expertise to bear at the Camouflage Development and Training Centre at Farnham Castle was the Cambridge zoologist Hugh Cott, author of the highly influential *Adaptive Coloration in Animals*, published in March 1940. For Cott, the practice of camouflage was not a natural activity for man – completely different from the unthinking genetic coloration of animals, which had evolved over millions of years – but a product of the First World War. He believed it was still in its infancy – 'a child suffering from arrested development' – and its importance and possibilities had yet to be fully appreciated by the British military establishment. Indeed, he fell out with them to the point that he resigned from his position on the Advisory Committee on Camouflage in April 1940. He was particularly critical of the dominance of artists in military camouflage, as he explained in a letter to Julian Huxley intended to be passed on to Professor Frederick Lindemann, Churchill's chief wartime scientific advisor.

'Camouflage research and application is at the present time largely dominated by artists,' wrote Cott, 'or in the hands of civil servants and regular officers, and in either case controlled by people lacking the necessary scientific training and having a profound ignorance of the fundamental biological and psycho-logical principles involved. This lack of appreciation of the scientific background of camouflage has led to the neglect, or misapplication, of such basic principles as countershading, dis-ruption, coincident pattern, deflection, and decoy. As a result much contemporary effort at camouflage has failed completely and is consistently failing to attain effectiveness.'

It was strong stuff, but Cott's criticisms were taken on board and his expertise appreciated at the Camouflage Development and Training Centre, where he lectured.

In 1941, Cott was transferred to North Africa, but there his reputation failed to impress his military superiors. In Cairo, Lieutenant-Colonel Geoffrey Barkas noted his academic work, but declared 'This has little application in the field where shit and bricks are all the materials you can get.'

Major Cott was appointed chief instructor at the Camouflage School at Helwan, Egypt. Julian Trevelyan, one of his students at Farnham Castle, visited him there and found the zoologist kept an entire menagerie of snakes, lizards and beetles in petrol cans around his camp.

Part of Cott's remit was to suggest the presence of vehicles and

☑ **Model of a German Messerschmitt Bf109E** fighter plane painted in a light shade on its underside to make it less visible when seen against the sky from below, and a dark shade on top to reduce its visibility from above. Zoologist Hugh Cott was very keen on promoting the use of such shading techniques in a military context.

weapons where there were none, allowing a build-up of real weaponry to occur elsewhere. One of the most ingenious of the deceptions he devised was the laying down of dummy shadows to suggest a line of tanks parked along desert roads.

Trevelyan visited one of grandest of the desert war camouflage schemes – an entire dummy railhead. 'No living man is there,' he said, 'but dummy men are grubbing in dummy swill-troughs, and dummy lorries are unloading dummy tanks, while a dummy engine puffs dummy smoke into the eyes of the enemy.'

Trevelyan had doubts about the effectiveness of this deception, however, when he and his colleagues were attacked near it by enemy aircraft. 'The planes have been over and shot at everything except the dummy railhead, which is unfortunate to say the least of it. They later paid it the compliment, I believe, of dropping a wooden bomb on it.'

Spreading the Word

Julian Trevelyan was one of several notable artist *camoufleurs* who passed through the Farnham Camouflage Development and Training Centre, including more traditional painters such as Frederick Gore and Edward Seago. Trevelyan was an avant-garde associate of Penrose, and with Stanley William Hayter they had set up an earlier, private Industrial Camouflage Research Unit in Bedford Square, London in 1939.

Trevelyan realized early on the psychological value of camouflage when he was working at the Industrial Camouflage Research Unit. 'People seemed to feel that the green stripes were a charm,' he said, 'that somehow brought them immunity from the unknown hazards of war; like the paper strips on the windows it made them feel that they had done their little bit, had invested in their small piece of 20th-century magic. In those early days it was easy to sell any kind of camouflage.'

The psychological boost of this illusion of security may have encouraged government efforts to promote camouflage in civil defence. But later publications endeavoured to get away from camouflage as a magic trick and stressed its practical necessity.

'Fougasse' was the pseudonym of the British cartoonist Cyril Kenneth Bird, famous for his 'Careless Talk Costs Lives' series of wartime public information posters. The French word *Fougasse* meant 'a small land mine which might or might not hit its mark'. He had served in the Royal Engineers in the First World War and was badly wounded at Gallipoli. By the beginning of the Second World War, he was art editor of *Punch* magazine and volunteered his services to the government. As a former Royal Engineer and an artist, he was attracted to the subject of camouflage, and illustrated an instructional booklet on the subject called *Hide & Seek*.

◢ *Camouflaging the Gun known as 'Winnie'*, inkwash by British Official War Artist Anthony Gross, 1941. A coastal defence gun near Dover is positioned beside a railway track under camouflage netting.

◢◢ *A 'Bell Gun Hide'*, one of the many applications of concealment netting devised by the British textile company Morton Sundour Fabrics Ltd (see also page 122).

▶ *RAF Regiment AA post*, watercolour by Eric Ravilious, 1942. An Official War Artist from 1940, Ravilious was killed in a flying accident off Iceland in 1942.

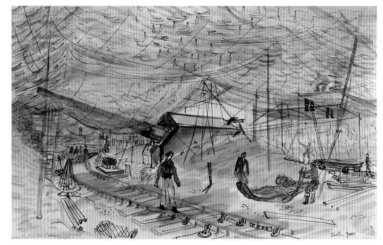

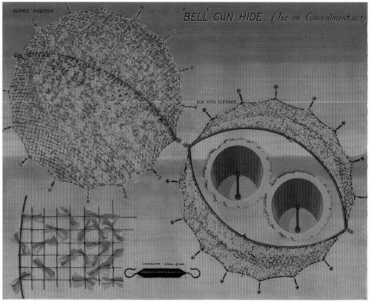

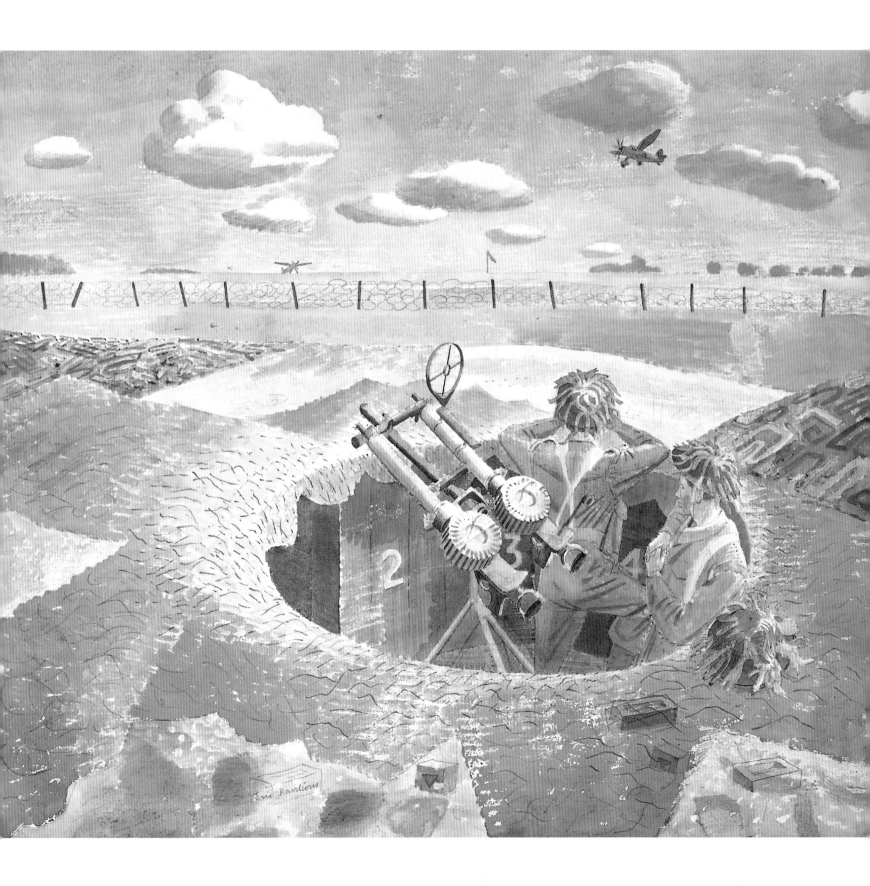

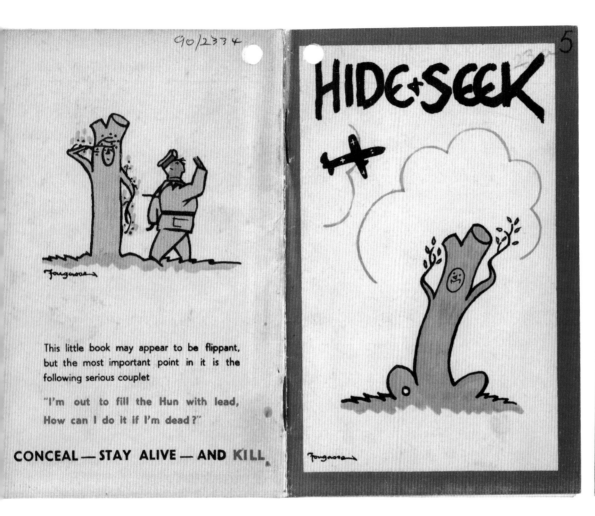

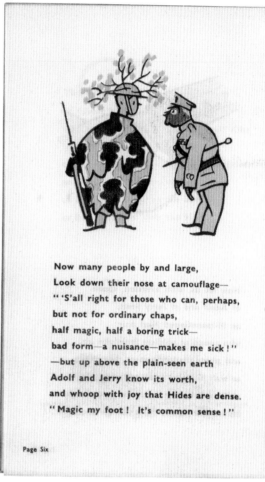

⚠ Pages from an instructional pamphlet on camouflage called *Hide & Seek*, illustrated by the British cartoonist Cyril Kenneth Bird. Under the pseudonym 'Fougasse', Bird found fame through his classic series of wartime public information posters bearing the message 'Careless Talk Costs Lives'. Produced for 5 Corps, this pamphlet tells in verse the cautionary tale of two soldier brothers called Albert and Thomas Hide.

Fougasse's booklet, produced for 5 Corps, tells the story in verse of two soldier brothers called Albert and Thomas Hide. In war, they are pursued by Adolf and Jerry Seek who 'snoop at soldiers from the air'. 'Now many people by and large,' said the story, 'look down their nose at camouflage – '"S'all right for those who can, perhaps, but not for ordinary chaps, half magic, half a boring trick – bad form – a nuisance – makes me sick!"'

But Tommy Hide takes it on board. 'The idea's immense!' he says 'Magic my foot! It's common sense.' His brother, Bert, however, ignores the demands of camouflage. 'A smart appearance,' he says, 'is ruined by a speck of dirt.' In the end, his bright buttons attract the bombs of the Nazi Seeks and, ironically, it is his brother Tommy who is killed in the blast.

The message is beautifully and amusingly told, but it is tough too, and the introduction by Lieutenant-General E.C.A. Schreiber

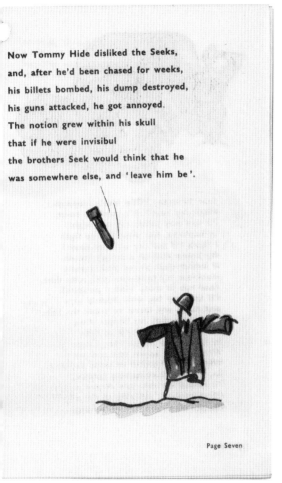

Now Tommy Hide disliked the Seeks,
and, after he'd been chased for weeks,
his billets bombed, his dump destroyed,
his guns attacked, he got annoyed.
The notion grew within his skull
that if he were invisibul
the brothers Seek would think that he
was somewhere else, and 'leave him be'.

Page Seven

Said Thomas: "The idea's immense!
Magic my foot! It's common sense.
I'll spit and polish day and night
in barracks, but when I've to fight
I think I'll dull my buttons down!
My boots shall be a muddy brown.
If British flesh shows pink, I must
black-out my handsome phiz with dust,
(and rub in more when I perspire).
I'll trim my hat with chicken wire
and twigs and leaves to break the line.
No longer shall my badges shine;
for though confusing it is right
to change my habits when I fight.
When not in action spit and polish!
When out for blood all brass abolish!
So, letting all equipment tarnish,
I'll spread my nets and thread my garnish,
(thick-centred, thinning to the edge),
and always drape it from a hedge

Page Eight

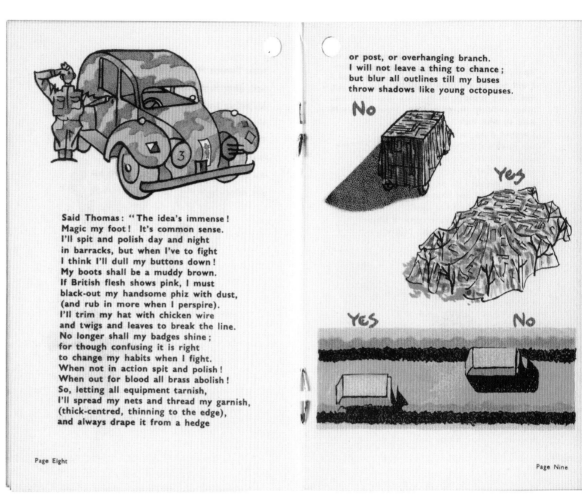

or post, or overhanging branch.
I will not leave a thing to chance;
but blur all outlines till my buses
throw shadows like young octopuses.

Page Nine

makes the point that the use of camouflage is not merely a passive process. It is also 'aggressive', he says. 'Concealment leads to deception of the enemy, and therefore to the attainment of surprise.' 'Surprise is a Weapon of Aggression,' concludes the booklet. 'It is NOT a passive covering-up.'

The US authorities employed cartoons to explain the complexities of camouflage. *100 Camouflage Questions and Answers* produced by the Engineer Section of the US First Air Force explained how to deceive enemy aerial photography, including images shot on infra-red film, which could penetrate obscuring weather conditions such as fog. The pamphlet had a step-by-step guide to texturing, showing how it could be applied to airfields and the roofs of military buildings. At the end was a list of seventeen other field manuals on various aspects of the subject available at each unit library. There was no excuse, at all, to be ignorant of camouflage.

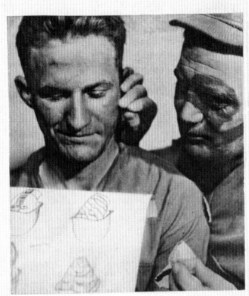

Soldiers do not have to be letter-perfect in this make-up, but simply follow a basic design.

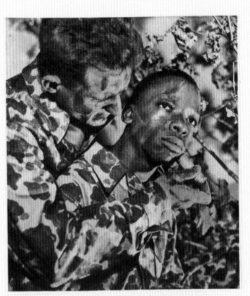

On dark skins, light green paint gives the best results. Application of a base coat is not necessary.

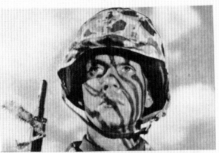

BAD. This design is too regular and hence does not sufficiently disrupt the symmetry of the soldier's face.

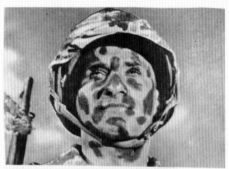

GOOD. Note the lines running vertical to the pupils, which effectively mask the eyes.

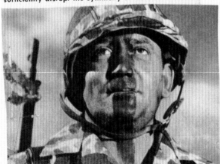

BAD. This solid band down the middle misses the eyes, the high lights of the cheekbones.

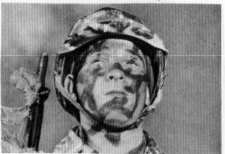

GOOD. This face pattern breaks the telltale shadow lines of the eyes, nose and mouth.

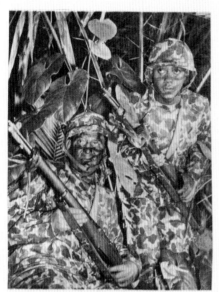

These outfits top anything even the Japs have devised for camouflage in tropical growth.

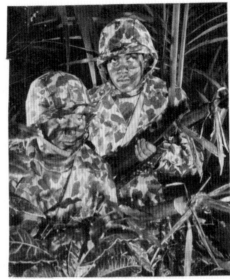

Soldiers improvise camouflage as they go along. Strips of palm fastened to these guns are good.

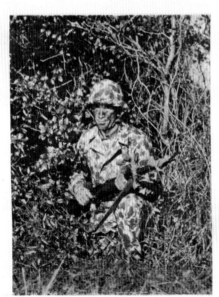

You'd have to get fully this close to see this soldier, whose battle dress blends perfectly with his background.

◁ **US wartime information flash cards** demonstrating the application and effectiveness of personal camouflage.

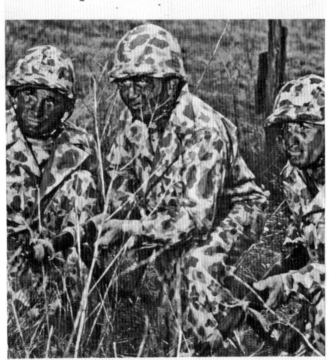

Their mothers might not recognize them, but neither may the enemy. Camouflage isn't expected to hide a man completely, but to make him harder for foe to see.

Camouflaging Industry

Camouflage attained a monumental scale in the Second World War. Total warfare engulfed civilian populations as aerial bombing raids became ever more destructive. Some believed that bombers alone could win the war by thoroughly destroying the infrastructure of an enemy nation. Fighter aircraft might have been in the frontline against the bombers, but it was camouflage that was deployed on the ground to fool enemy pilots and aerial reconnaissance photographers. Factory roofs were painted to look like housing estates, grass-covered airfields were criss-crossed with tar strips to look like hedgerows, railway stations were smothered in netting and foliage, train tracks painted to look like roads. It was a monumental task – to camouflage a whole nation.

One British Camouflage Committee memorandum of 1943 looked at finding cheap methods to darken factory buildings.

◤ *Men Fixing Feathered Netting over a Factory*, watercolour by Cedric John Kennedy, 1942. Two men roll out camouflage material over a net framework suspended above a factory.

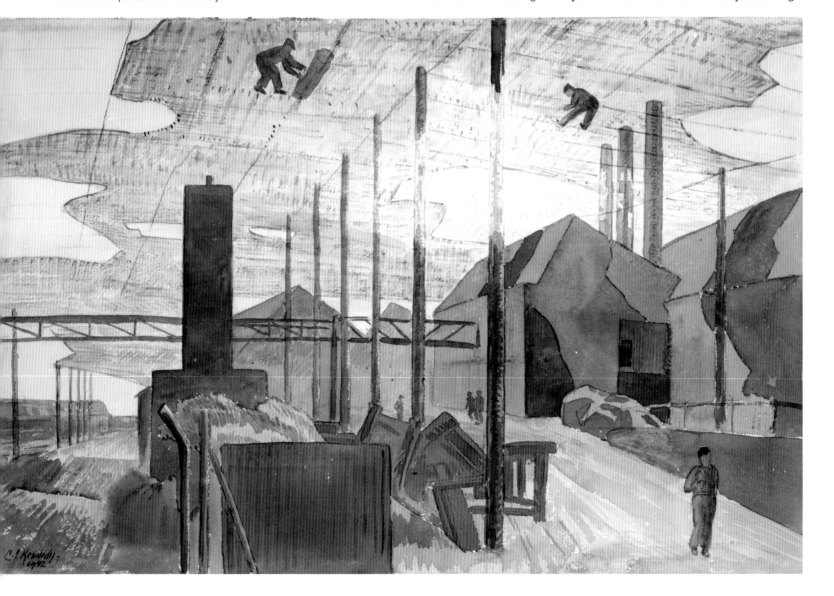

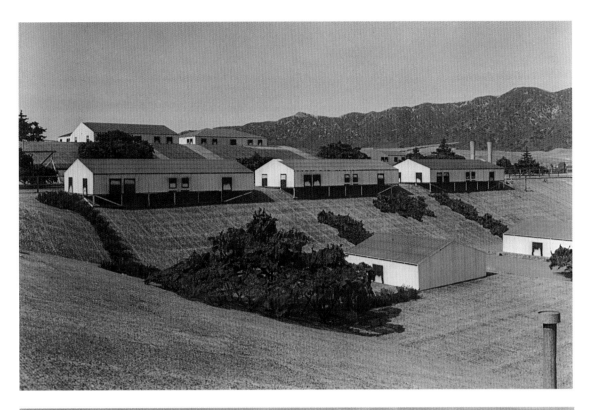

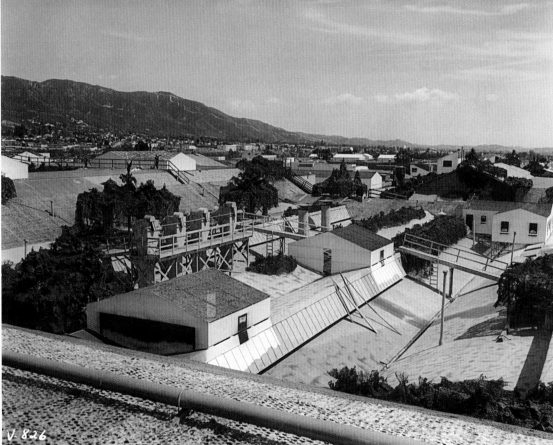

▶ **Aerial views of Lockheed aircraft-making factory** in Burbank, California, hidden under a vast canopy of shrubs, grass and fake houses.

V-826

'As so many buildings are now made of materials that are pale in tone,' it said, 'galvanized iron, concrete, asbestos sheeting, etc – it is of great importance to find a cheap, rapid and effective method of darkening such buildings.'

One of the materials they selected was sludge oil – the dirty residue from processing crude oil or fuel oil. The sludge oil was emulsified with water and then mixed with other waste material such as coke grit and waste slaked lime sludge, to help it dry and prevent shine. This mixture was then applied to the tops of buildings with long-handled brushes. 'The lasting qualities of sludge oil seem good,' concluded the Committee.

An alternative camouflage scheme for factories had been suggested by an Air Raid Precautions Handbook of 1939 entitled *Camouflage of Large Installations*. This gave two variants for painting a spread of factory roofs. One was an imitative pattern in which local colours such as tile red, slate grey, buff ground, black shadows and green grass were applied to the top of the factory in order to make it look like nearby housing; the other variant was to use the same colours but in a random disruptive pattern. Artist Colin Moss produced a series of paintings recording the extraordinary spectacle of such camouflaged buildings (overleaf).

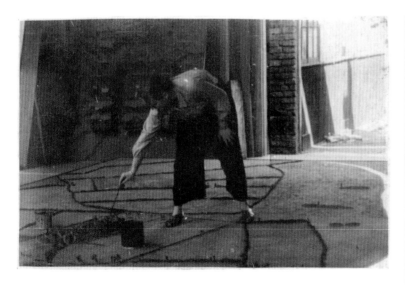

◪ **A civilian worker paints a model of a camouflage scheme**, *c*. 1940, in Leamington Spa, central England, home to the Civil Defence Camouflage Establishment. Designs were prepared for testing in a hall known as 'the Rink', which had a special viewing balcony.

▶ **Painting camouflage materials** in the workshop at Leamington Spa.

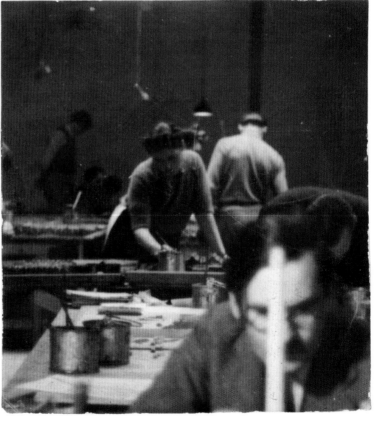

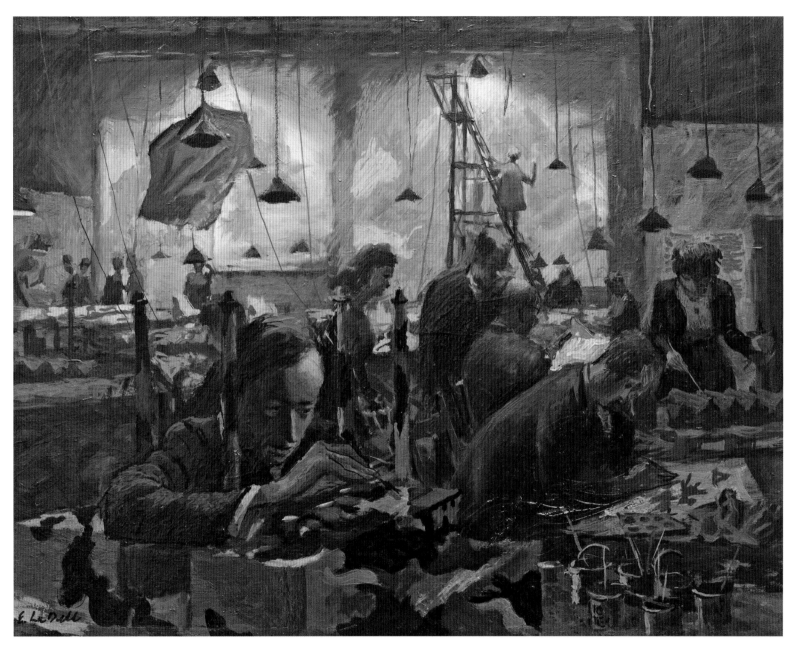

◤ *The Camouflage Workshop*,
oil on panel by Edwin La Dell, 1940.
These civilian *camoufleurs* are shown
at work in Leamington Spa. Sections
of finished camouflage are hung from
the ceiling and could be checked from
the viewing balcony.

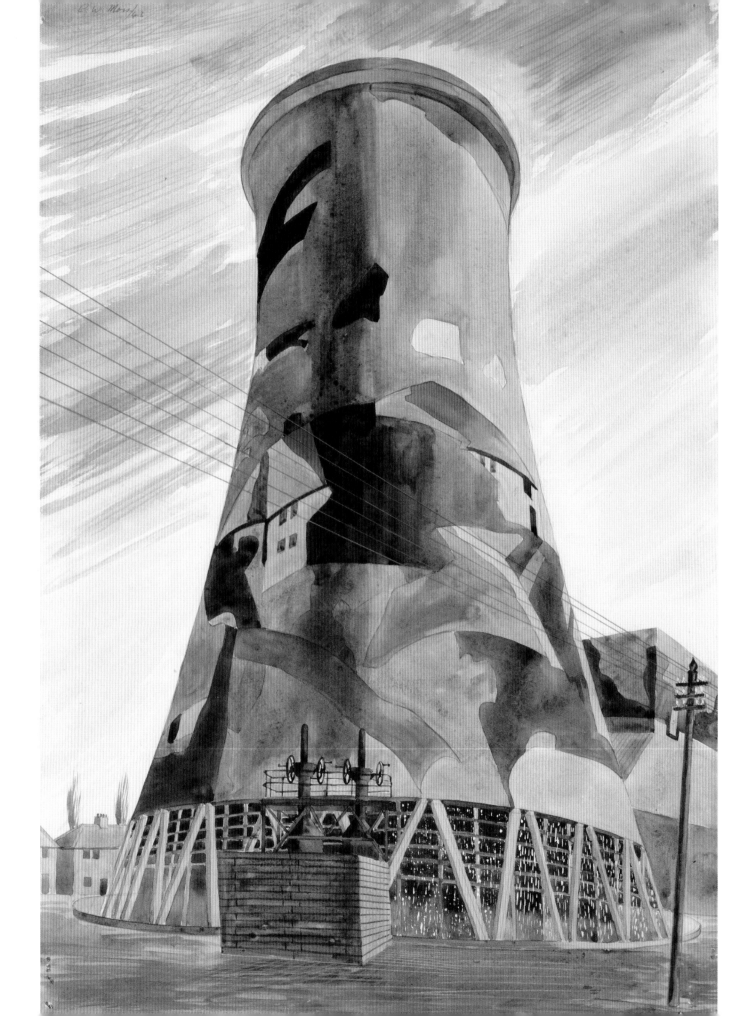

◄ *The Big Tower, Camouflaged,* watercolour by Colin Moss, 1943. This water tower at Stonebridge Park Power Station, near Wembley in London, was disguised with images of houses and a disruptive pattern painted by Moss and other artists employed by the Ministry of Home Security's Camouflage Directorate.

▶ *A Camouflage Scheme in Progress*, watercolour by Colin Moss, 1943. Here Moss depicts a team of artists painting camouflage on the roof of a building.

◄ *Camouflaged Cooling-Towers*, watercolour by Colin Moss, 1943.

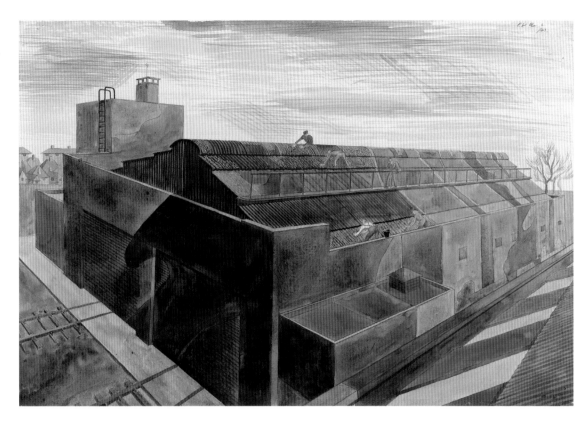

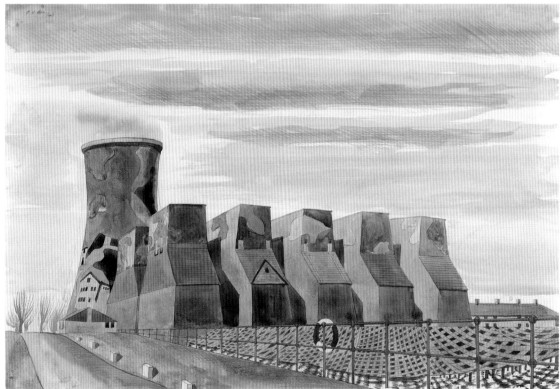

Oil installations were a prime target for German bombers and one report produced by Captain Ronald Smith of the Royal Engineers G.III camouflage section gave a detailed assessment of how to disguise them.

'Half an hour's flight over the area puts the camouflage officer on the right track and the rough camouflage scheme evolves,' said Smith. 'Photographs should be taken from every angle and later studied carefully.'

A large-scale drawing illustrating the scheme was then drawn up. This was followed by a thorough costing of the project. Once approval had been given, the work could begin. Some usual camouflage materials could not be employed. 'For example, the use of string netting is forbidden because of the fire danger,' advised Smith, 'and non-combustible substitutes are scarce.'

Ideally, the *camoufleur* aimed to apply a disruptive pattern using substances derived from the products of the oil installation, such as bitumen, good for shadow effects, or another distillate residue, which when used with local clay, blended to form an excellent sand-coloured paint.

Painting equipment was simple, and included brushes made out of rope strands bound by scrap tin. Experience had taught Captain Smith that one painter could cover approximately 1200 square feet (110 square metres) per day. Ground patterning

British Standard Camouflage Colour	Notes
SHADE No. 11A	
SHADE No. 11B	
SHADE No. 12	

B.S. 987C : 1942   Plate Three

◤ ▷ **Swatches showing approved** colours and paint colour charts were among the tools of the trade of camouflage artists. Even before the outbreak of war, the British Air Ministry had held discussions with the National Paint Federation in 1939, as a result of which a type of camouflage paint was manufactured in fourteen colours and shades.

◀ **'Camouflage Colours' booklet** produced by the British Standards Institute, September 1942, with pages of colour charts. These were issued to camouflage officers and to firms producing camouflage materials to ensure that correct colours were used.

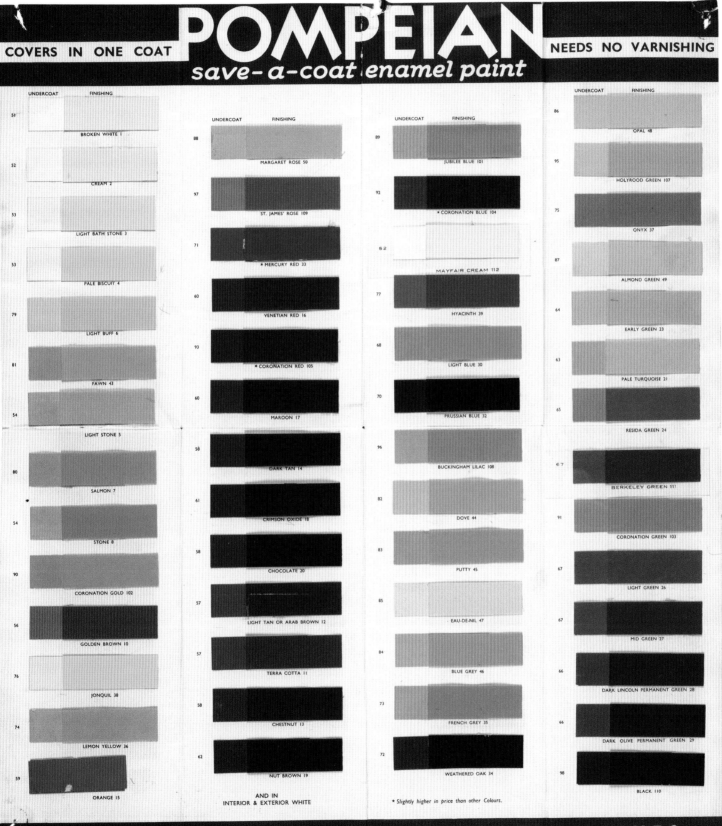

POMPEIAN
save-a-coat enamel paint

COVERS IN ONE COAT

NEEDS NO VARNISHING

UNDERCOAT	FINISHING

51 BROKEN WHITE 1

52 CREAM 2

53 LIGHT BATH STONE 3

53 PALE BISCUIT 4

79 LIGHT BUFF 6

81 FAWN 43

54 LIGHT STONE 5

80 SALMON 7

54 STONE 8

90 CORONATION GOLD 102

56 GOLDEN BROWN 10

76 JONQUIL 38

74 LEMON YELLOW 36

59 ORANGE 15

88 MARGARET ROSE 50

97 ST. JAMES' ROSE 109

71 * MERCURY RED 33

60 VENETIAN RED 16

93 * CORONATION RED 105

60 MAROON 17

58 DARK TAN 14

61 CRIMSON OXIDE 18

58 CHOCOLATE 20

57 LIGHT TAN OR ARAB BROWN 12

57 TERRA COTTA 11

58 CHESTNUT 13

62 NUT BROWN 19

AND IN
INTERIOR & EXTERIOR WHITE

89 JUBILEE BLUE 101

92 * CORONATION BLUE 104

52 MAYFAIR CREAM 112

77 HYACINTH 39

68 LIGHT BLUE 30

70 PRUSSIAN BLUE 32

96 BUCKINGHAM LILAC 108

82 DOVE 44

83 PUTTY 45

85 EAU-DE-NIL 47

84 BLUE GREY 46

73 FRENCH GREY 35

72 WEATHERED OAK 34

* Slightly higher in price than other Colours.

UNDERCOAT	FINISHING

86 OPAL 48

95 HOLYROOD GREEN 107

75 ONYX 37

87 ALMOND GREEN 49

64 EARLY GREEN 23

63 PALE TURQUOISE 21

65 RESIDA GREEN 24

67 BERKELEY GREEN 111

91 CORONATION GREEN 103

67 LIGHT GREEN 26

67 MID GREEN 27

66 DARK LINCOLN PERMANENT GREEN 28

66 DARK OLIVE PERMANENT GREEN 29

98 BLACK 110

NO COMPLAINTS WITH BERGER PAINTS

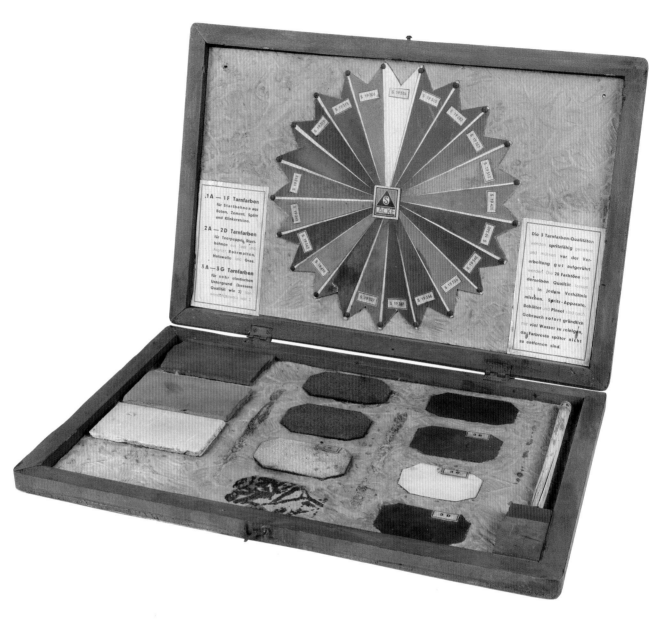

⬛ German paint sample case
for camouflaging aircraft runways.
The underside of the lid shows a 'dial'
of twenty prescribed camouflage
colours. The paint samples on the left
are suitable for runways constructed of
concrete, aggregate, clinker or cement.
Those in the centre are for bitumen,
asphalt, wood-wool or grass. Those on
the right are for more elastic surfaces.

would be applied first, then representations of buildings in an overall disruptive pattern of dark and light shapes that masked the entire area.

To cover the ground, Captain Smith recommended that 'a lasting pattern can be produced by sprayed bitumen raked into a rough textured surface with white, sharp river sand as the contrasting colour of the pattern. Should the area include storage tanks, roofs and shadows will merge most successfully into the pattern by geometric disruptive painting.'

To disguise white smoke coming out of refinery chimneys, it was suggested that the fuel be altered to produce a darker smoke. As for nearby water, a mixture of bitumized earth could be spread across its surface to dull its reflectiveness.

As Germany suffered from the increasing intensity of Allied bombing raids, *camoufleurs* there also developed camouflage to hide industrial and urban centres. Smoke-screens had been used

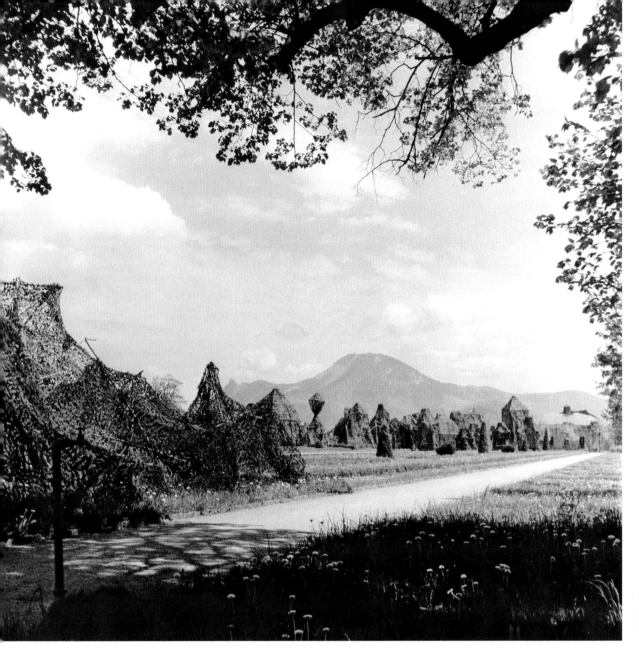

◁ **Camouflage netting** covers statues and features in the grounds of Schloss Linderhof, Germany, in an attempt to thwart Allied reconnaissance. Photograph by Lee Miller, 1945.

early on in the war but had proved unpopular with factory workers who complained about the acrid, chemically-generated fumes. Building on their achievements in the First World War, the Germans also pursued large structural schemes rather than rely on paint. One synthetic rubber plant in the Ruhr was placed under a massive spread of wire netting interwoven with tufts of glass wool. This was then repainted to match the colours of the changing seasons. Such efforts were very demanding of manpower and materials. As an alternative, an entire decoy factory was built a few miles away, complete with fake buildings and streets – though in the event this did not attract a single Allied bomb.

In the final years of the war, German *camoufleurs* became increasingly desperate and tried to mask their factories by pretending they were already abandoned mounds of rubble. Some factories were even rebuilt inside the blasted shells of their old buildings. Among the most ambitious German camouflage

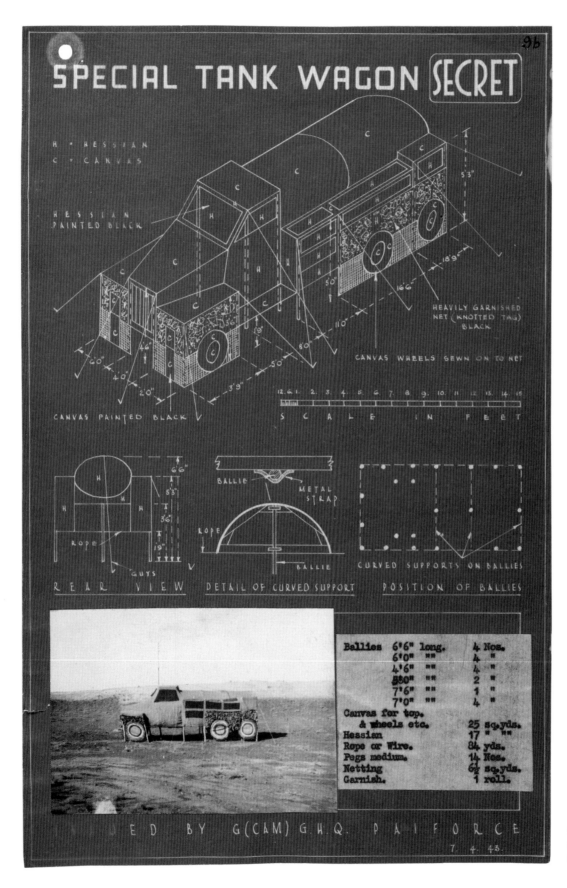

◀ **Blueprint for creating a dummy truck.** The Allied production of decoy military vehicles was a vital weapon against German aerial reconnaissance.

schemes were entire lakes covered with platforms so as to appear as solid land. Such projects were only possible because of the use of slave workers.

Without access to forced labour, the Allies had to rely on their ingenuity. Allied camouflage experts devoted part of their time to the creation of decoys. This was pursued throughout the war. A letter kept in the papers of Major Denys Pavitt of the Camouflage Development and Training Centre describes the testing of dummy tanks at Skipsea on the east coast of England in March 1942:

'At first sight the dummy tanks were indistinguishable from the real article,' said the report, 'and the difference was not noted until pilots had dived over them, and were finishing their attacks. Then, however, sufficient points of identification were noted to prevent pilots being deceived a second time by a similar set-up.

'The general opinion is that the tracks and camouflage were too light in colour, and the pilots suggest that a much darker tone on the upper surface and dark brown or even black on the tracks would make for greater conviction.'

Two more years of such practical experimentation meant that the industry of producing dummy weapons and equipment was near perfect when the time came for its greatest test. Operation Fortitude was the name given to the task of convincing German intelligence that an entire army group was based in south-east England under the command of US General George S. Patton, and was intending to invade at the Pas de Calais rather than what was to be the actual landing area in Normandy. This army did not exist.

False oil storage tanks, landing jetties, and anti-aircraft emplacements were built. Dummy landing craft were made out of canvas stretched over tubular steel frames and mixed with real landing craft to give the impression of an invasion fleet moored far away from the real one. Inflatable rubber Sherman tanks stood in fields, while decoy aircraft were made out of painted sections of wood bolted together. Many of the people involved in creating these illusions were craftsmen from British film studios working alongside military camouflage experts. As well as visual trickery, the whole operation was supported by radio and radar deception. So successful was the ruse that even after the Allied landings at Normandy, Hitler still believed the main attack would come at the Pas de Calais, where his forces remained at their strongest.

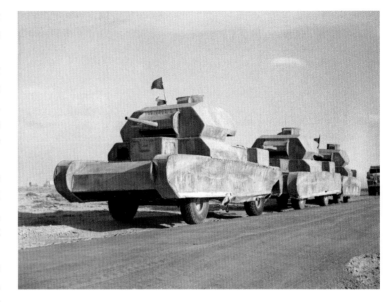

◢ **British trucks disguised as dummy tanks** in North Africa. The use of decoy vehicles helped mislead the Germans as to where the next major Allied offensive was coming from. They were deployed extensively during the El Alamein campaign in 1942.

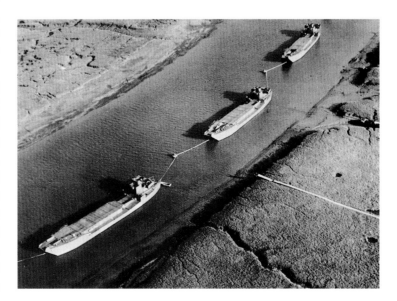

◢ **Dummy landing craft** moored in an English river, part of the mammoth deception effort in the summer of 1944 that successfully tricked the Germans into thinking that the Allied invasion of France was to come at the Pas de Calais rather than Normandy. An entirely false army was located far from the real invasion force.

Camouflage for Every Soldier

As the war progressed, it was realized that though specialized units of *camoufleurs* had their role to play in major strategic camouflage schemes, the importance of camouflage on the field of battle was something that every soldier had to understand. A pamphlet issued by British GHQ in the Middle East in July 1941 tackled this point head on.

'It is true that the camouflage of large installations is a highly specialized craft,' said the pamphlet. 'The concealment of armies in the field is a totally different proposition. It is a vast problem because every single member of the army contributes to it every day in the normal course of his work and life....

'It is believed that study of this book, coupled with a little imagination, will make any intelligent officer or NCO a reliable instructor and supervisor of practical camouflage work for his unit in the field.'

▼ *Coast Defence Battle*, oil on canvas, by Barnett Freedman, September 1940. Freedman was an Official War Artist, first with the British Expeditionary Force in France, then with the Admiralty until 1946.

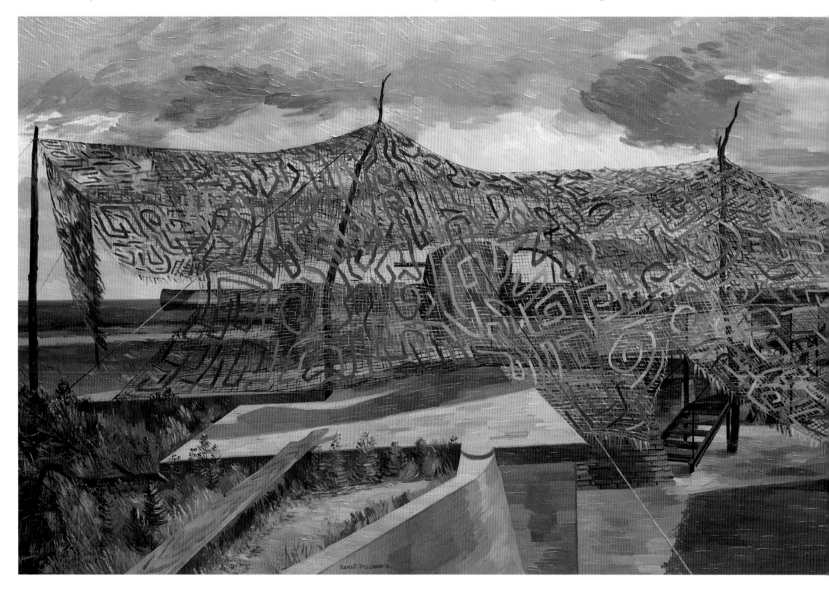

The pamphlet covered the basics of camouflage theory and attempted to convey exactly what an enemy reconnaissance pilot would be looking for on the ground. It declared that the main adversaries were the eye and above all the lens, which registered the troops' presence and activities in shades of black, white and grey. The pamphlet analysed what made objects appear light or dark and how texture and colour could affect their appearance. Positioning was all-important. Well-annotated photographs demonstrated how features that looked light to an airman were those with smooth and level surfaces, such as roads, sunlit rooftops, and areas where grass or soil had been flattened by movement.

In the harsh environment of desert warfare, many troops put their faith in erecting camouflage nets over their positions. The pamphlet insisted that this possessed no magic in itself. 'Throughout the army there are thousands upon thousands of

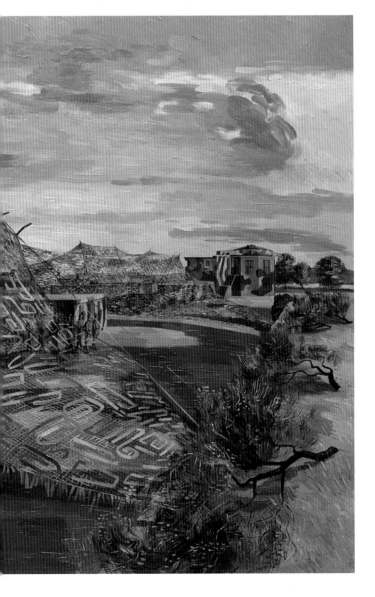

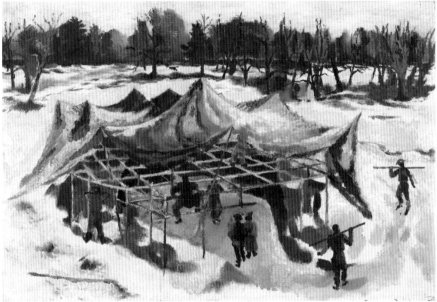

◩ *A Covering For a Gunsite*, oil on panel, by Albert Richards, 1942. Richards depicts British soldiers at work in a clearing, assembling a framework which is partially covered in tarpaulins. He was an amateur artist and a paratrooper who was appointed as an Official War Artist in 1944, ten months before his death aged 25.

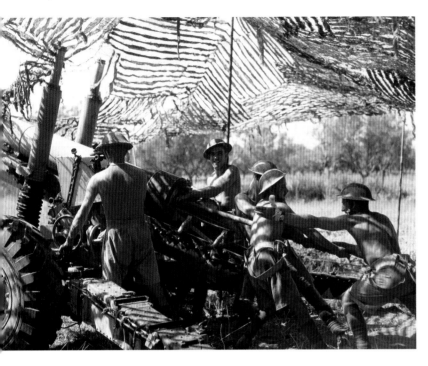

people who evidently believe that an ungarnished large-mesh net makes their trench or their vehicle invisible. It does not. If a British eye can see slap through it, so can a German or Italian eye. A large-mesh net with no garnish is about as useful as an application of vanishing cream. The garnish may be regulation strip, or torn up hessian, or rags or clumps of vegetation or twigs of branches. The net by itself is useless.'

The pamphlet also pricked the idea that painting a disruptive pattern on a tank would offer it magic protection in a desert landscape. 'The designs painted on the tanks may be excellent camouflage at ground level... [but] they are certainly not good camouflage against aerial observation in this particular setting.' Their patterns stood out all too clearly against a plain light-coloured ground.

◤ **British gunners of the** Shropshire Yeomanry in Italy in action with a 5.5-inch howitzer under camouflage netting.

◨ **Different concealment nettings**. This watercolour drawing was produced by Morton Sundour Fabrics Ltd, a British textile firm which switched from producing furniture fabrics to making camouflage materials during the Second World War. The 'Square Type' net (top left) was used by all branches of the forces, and was even claimed to be effective against infra-red photography.

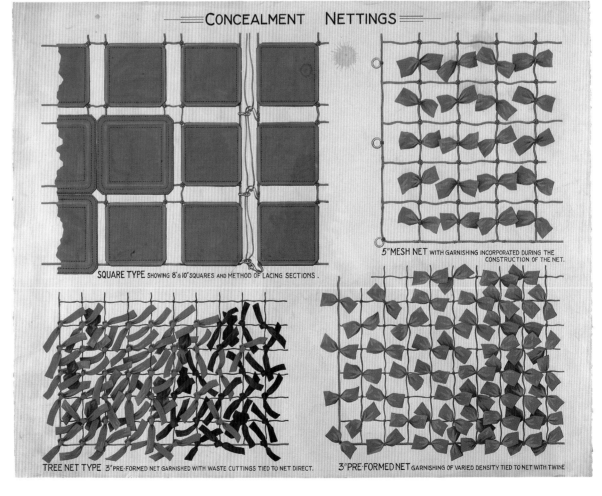

CONCEALMENT NETTINGS

SQUARE TYPE SHOWING 8" & 10" SQUARES AND METHOD OF LACING SECTIONS.

5" MESH NET WITH GARNISHING INCORPORATED DURING THE CONSTRUCTION OF THE NET.

TREE NET TYPE 3" PRE-FORMED NET GARNISHED WITH WASTE CUTTINGS TIED TO NET DIRECT.

3" PRE-FORMED NET GARNISHING OF VARIED DENSITY TIED TO NET WITH TWINE

ARTILLERY NETS

Camouflage nets should, ideally, be garnished to suit each individual site. In practice it is necessary to garnish nets so that they fit in fairly well on various normal backgrounds, but these nets must be adapted on the site to match in with the immediate background.

PATCHES whether of solid scrim or garnishing strip are intended to obscure and break up the shape of the object or area to be concealed. They should usually be large and very ragged in shape. Bow Tie or Knot garnish gives texture to the net. Spaces between patches on the area of net giving cover should be fully garnished with knots. Knot garnish round outer edges of patches is intended to soften cast shadow and to merge with background. So areas of knots should thin out towards a ragged outer edge.

PATCHES of solid Scrim.

Materials : Hessian scrim (6-oz. or 8-oz.) cut from the roll or from sheets hessian 12-ft. × 20-ft. If hessian is not available in this form use w/s latrine canvas, sandbags, tentage, cotton scrim, or any salvage material. Coarse rough textured material is preferable.

Cutting : Each patch should be cut (or made up) at least ¼ larger than the area it is to cover when attached to the net.

Sew edges of patch to net along lines of mesh. Avoid sewing diagonally across net.

Pucker up loose material in centre of patch and tie down to net at approximately three feet intervals with lengths of garnish strip.

Fig.1 Stitching, Puckering and Tying down.

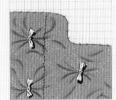

PATCHES of Garnishing strip.

Alternatively, patch areas may be garnished with garnishing strip. It is convenient to make up each patch area with 2-ft. square units, each unit garnished as in Fig. 2.

Fig.2 Strip garnishing for a 2-ft. unit.

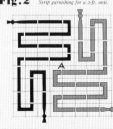

Thread two 13-ft. lengths of garnishing strip into the net, commencing at "A" so that every hole in the mesh is filled. Fig. 2 does not indicate method of CORNERING which should be the "Box" method as in Fig. 3.

Fig.3 Cornering.

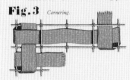

Garnish strip should lie flat and be tied with a firm knot at each end. Garnish must be slack to allow for stretching of the net.

BOW TIE Garnishing.

A 5-in. length of garnishing strip is fastened across a knot in the net with string by a simple reef knot.

Fig.4 Bow Tie Garnishing.

KNOT Garnishing.

Alternatively, a 10-in. length of garnishing strip is tied tightly across a knot in the mesh.

Fig.5 Knot Garnishing.

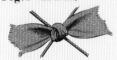

Whenever possible garnish by the bow tie method. It is slower, but less material is used so that the net weighs less. It has a better appearance and weathers better.

ARRANGEMENT

The diagrams in the next column are a guide for general purpose garnishing.

Patches of Hessian, or similar material, or flat strip garnishing with a few knots tied over the strip.

Bow tie (or knot) garnish tied across every knot in the mesh of the net.

Bow tie (or knot) garnish tied across every alternate knot in the mesh of the net.

GARNISHING Diagrams

If the same pattern is used on all nets of one Troop of guns, each net must have the laced slit placed at a different side.

35' × 35' Artillery Net.   Diagram No. 27.

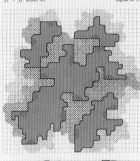

35' × 17' Extension Net.   Diagram No. 28.

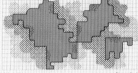

29' × 29' Artillery Net. Diagram No. 31.

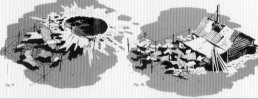

29' × 14' Extension Net. Diagram No. 32.

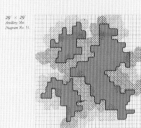

35' × 35' Net. Diagram No. 29.

An arrangement of 2-ft. square units of flat strip garnish on patch areas.

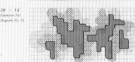
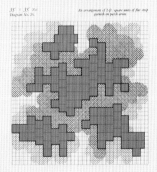

IN THE FIELD

CRASH ACTION. Do not use Artillery frame. Shield cover must be in position. If necessary use net as a drape to break up shape of gun and limber to obliterate shine.

NORMAL DEPLOYMENT including A/Tk role in a prepared defensive position. Avoid siting on featureless ground, link up with some existing feature. When digging in, full camouflage equipment (Arty. frame, with Posts, Brackets Sleeve and Extensions) should be erected as a LOW mounded cover as soon as possible. All spoil and light reflecting surfaces under the cover should be darkened down. Garnishing must be adapted to match the immediate background. Foliage (other than flat leaved), brushwood, Army or domestic salvage, or any other local material may be used. Fig. 9 shews a patch net designed to match the pattern of a bomb crater. Fig. 10 shews split sandbags and domestic salvage arranged on net as a lean-to roof, and rubbish.

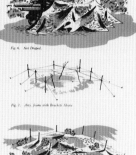

Fig. 6. Net Draped.

Fig. 7. Arty. frame with Brackets Sleeve.

Fig. 8. Completed mound.

SPECIAL COVERS patches designed for individual sites.

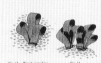

Fig. 9.   Fig. 10.

SHIELD COVERS

In the field (N. Europe) all gun shields must be covered to prevent shine, which reveals position to low oblique air view.

SHAPE FORMER (detachable). An iron bar bent to a low irregular shape fitted with clamps for attachment to shield.

SHIELD COVER. A Piece of hessian is cut to hang over front of shield supported by a bar which fits over shape former. Cut with an irregular margin to hang over sides and base of shield. Paint very DARK BROWN with a non-oil paint (S.C.C. No. 1A).

BUNCH GARNISHING. 2-ft. lengths of strip to be bunched as Fig. 13, and sewn to cover approximately 9-ins. apart. Larger bunches to be sewn to top edges of cover - Fig. 14.

CULLACORTS COVER. Feathered wire netting cut to an irregular shape so that it overlaps edges of shield. Cut, and twist at edges and wire twisted pieces on to front of cover so that they cast shadows on the cover. See Fig. 15.

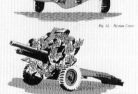

Fig. 11. Shape Former.

Fig. 12. Hessian Cover.

Fig. 13. Bunch garnishing.   Fig. 14.   Fig. 15. Cullacorts.

COLOUR proportions vary with the time of year and place.

SOLID SCRIM patches should be darker than the background. Colour areas should be large, if possible each patch one colour throughout.

FLAT GARNISH patches. Colour area should cover three or more 2-ft. square units.

BOW TIES (or Knots) Colours should be used indiscriminately.

ADD local colour to match in with the background. Use light colours with discretion.

NETS. Light coloured nets should not be garnished for use in N. Europe. If net is badly faded, darken ungarnished areas with paint, creosote, or sump oil.

BUNCH GARNISH (For Shield Covers). Divide cover into five or six irregular areas, most areas to be bunched with light garnish, a few with dark garnish.

◤ Instructional poster for disguising artillery positions with camouflage netting, issued by the British War Office in 1942.

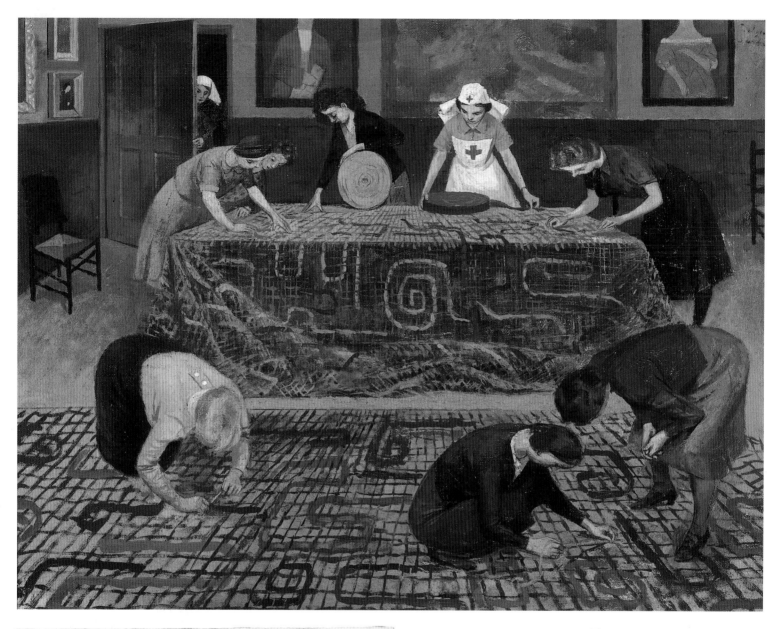

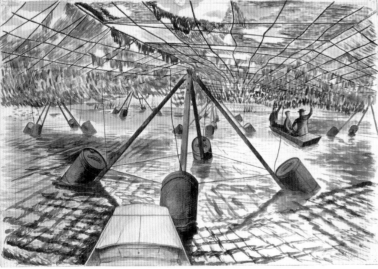

◭ Convalescent Nurses Making Camouflage Nets, oil painting by Evelyn Dunbar, 1941. Nurses evacuated from London are being involved in this valuable work in Wales.

◀ Experimental Camouflage: Inspecting Camouflage Nets Suspended over Water to Conceal it from the Air, drawing and watercolour by Eric Hall. The netting garnish is being inspected by a team of *camoufleurs* in a boat.

▶ Women attach cloth garnish to camouflage netting in an old school building in London, 1943, one of the many depots of the Women's Voluntary Service engaged in this work, which involved large numbers of civilian helpers.

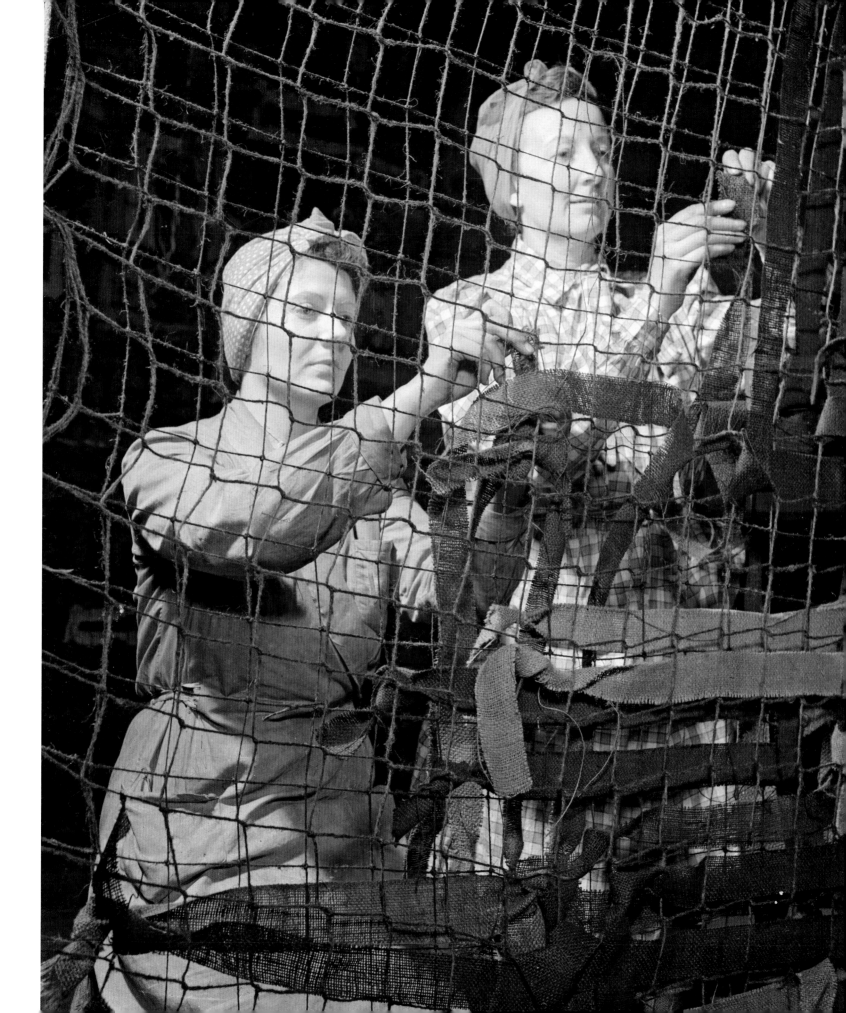

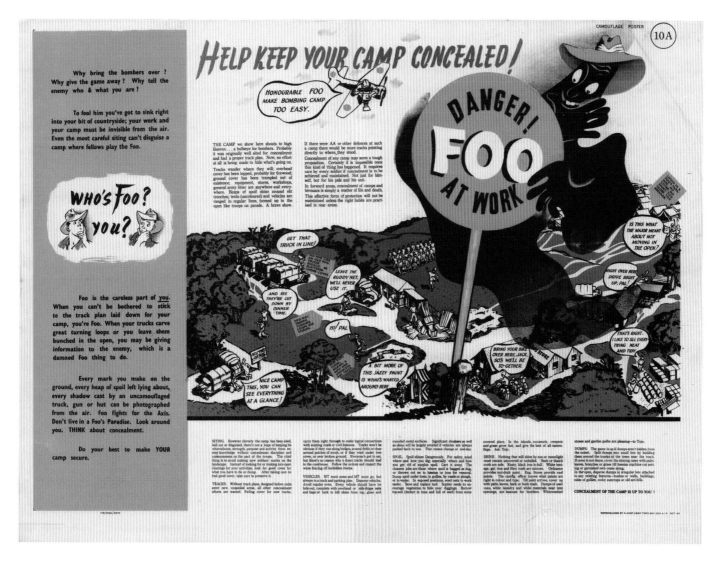

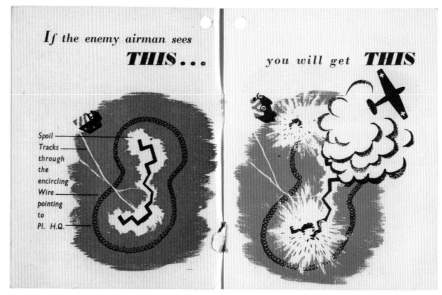

⬛ **Australian poster** giving advice to soldiers on how to conceal a camp.

▶ *Surprise: The First Principle of Attack*. British instructional leaflet revealing how tracks around a camp can reveal the presence of a position to the enemy above.

Other pamphlets also stressed the importance of how every soldier bore a responsibility for maintaining the effective camouflage of a position. *Notes on Camouflage in the BEF* (British Expeditionary Force) said that disguised tracks around a military base must be adhered to. 'The first man therefore to be careless or lazy enough to take a short cut, may be responsible for the shells or bombs which will inevitably fall on the spot.' This even extended to the path to and from camp latrines. Wire at night was recommended as a guide to soldiers stumbling about in the dark to relieve themselves.

How to make camouflage easily understood by the ordinary soldier was a theme returned to at the end of the war in a series of pamphlets on visual training for military instructors called *VIZ*. In the first issue in February 1945, General Sir Harold Franklyn, Commander-in-Chief of the Home Forces, looked to the future and said that camouflage during the war 'has been left to the specialists and has not been accepted as a normal Army training responsibility. The present system might well break down at the end of the war when the specialists return to their civil occupations. Unless we take steps now to integrate the subject thoroughly in army training there is a possibility that much of the valuable experience gained in this war will be wasted.'

The Commandant of the Camouflage Development and Training Centre agreed and added his own radical proposal in *VIZ*. 'It is clear that the word 'camouflage' should be avoided in early training,' he said. 'The recruit can learn all he needs to know about camouflage painlessly without ever being given the impression that he is learning a specialist subject. The simple reasons why things are recognized, the forms of observation to which recognition must be denied must be explained, and some suggestions on the factors affecting the priority which should be given to avoidance of recognition, must be given.'

The Commandant wanted camouflage training to be accepted as a basic skill alongside physical training. He considered it misleading to separate fieldcraft and camouflage, because camouflage was essential to good fieldcraft, just as being physically fit was essential. The message was clear. Camouflage was fundamental to modern warfare and every single recruit should absorb it along with square-bashing.

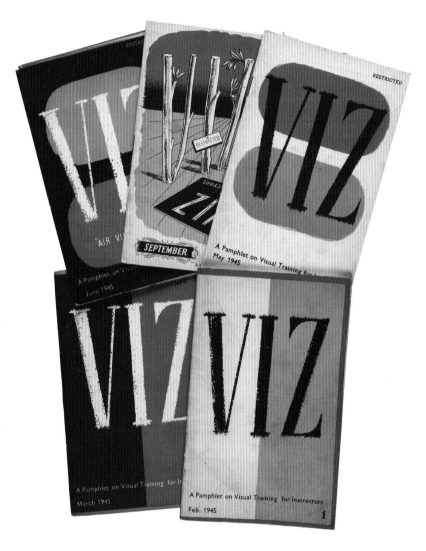

▶ **Pages from *VIZ***, a British Army journal devoted to all aspects of visual training, including camouflage, among soldiers.

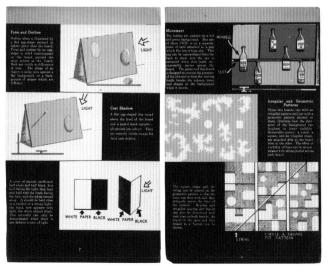

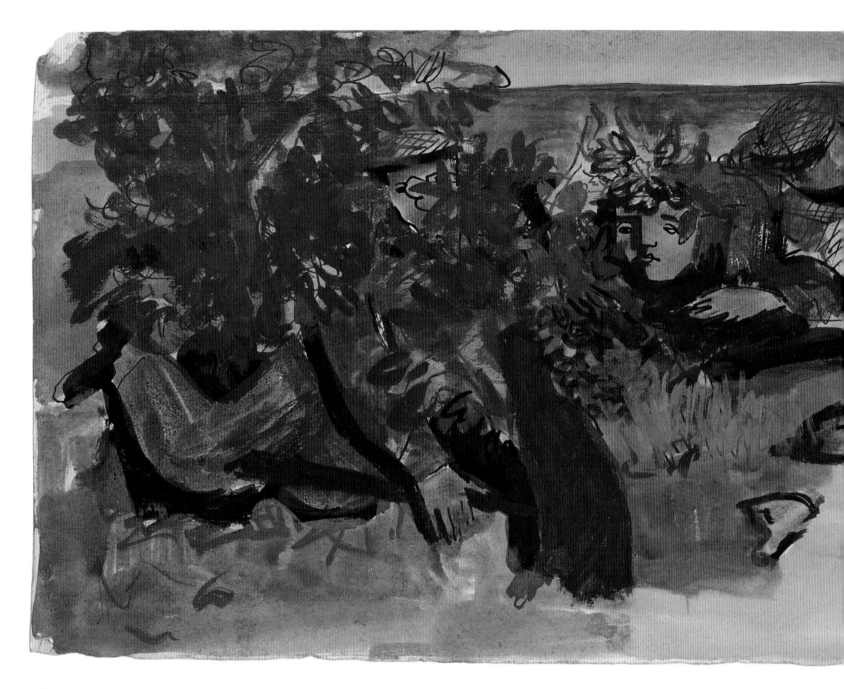

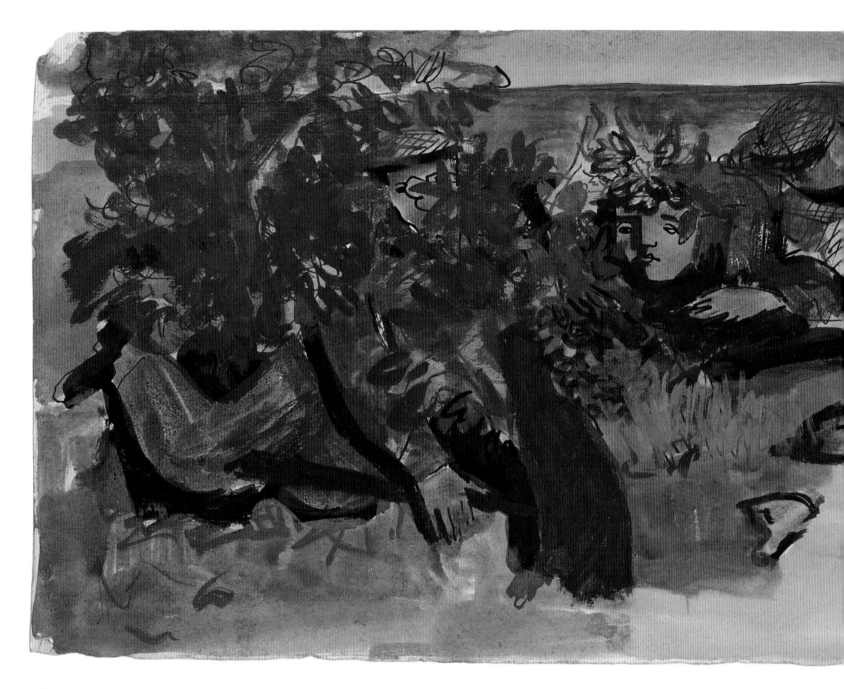 *Camouflaged Soldiers*, gouache on paper, by William Scott, 1943. Scott served with the British Royal Engineers for nearly four years from 1942.

Camouflage Uniforms

As in the First World War, the vast majority of soldiers entered battle wearing single-colour combat uniforms. The British and Americans usually wore khaki or green, while the Germans wore grey. But as the war progressed, specialist units evolved and they tended to wear specially designed clothing.

In Britain, in 1941, paratroopers were issued the Denison Smock, a heavy-duty, waterproof item covered with a simple large brush-stroke-style camouflage pattern of light green with ragged areas of dark green and chocolate brown printed on top of it. This brush-stroke design may well have been the origin of a similar motif still used in today's British Army disruptive pattern material or DPM (see pages 4–5). The paratrooper smock was named after its designer Captain Denison, who served with a camouflage unit commanded by the renowned stage designer Oliver Messel. Camouflage one-piece suits were worn by British tank crews and Allied agents parachuted into occupied territory. But on the whole, camouflage clothing remained a marginal aspect of British combat dress.

It was a similar story in the US Army. Most American troops wore a shade of green, in particular the predominant olive drab. Camouflage overalls were first issued to the US Marines in 1943 in the Pacific War. These proved highly unpopular, being too hot and awkward for jungle warfare, and they were superseded by a

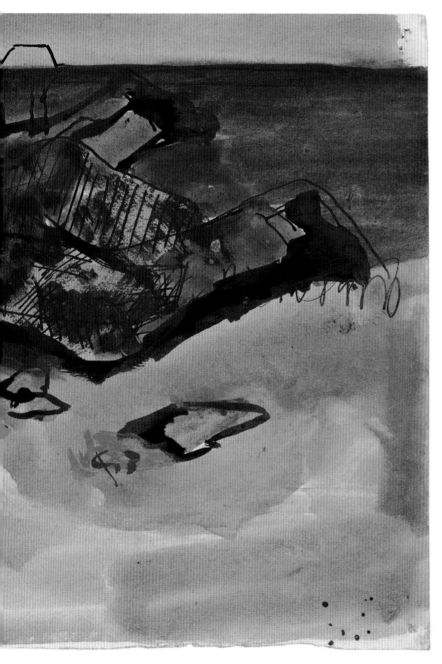

▶ *Troops Crossing a Jungle Stream*, watercolour on paper by Thomas Barclay Hennell, 1945–46. This jungle scene was painted in Burma.

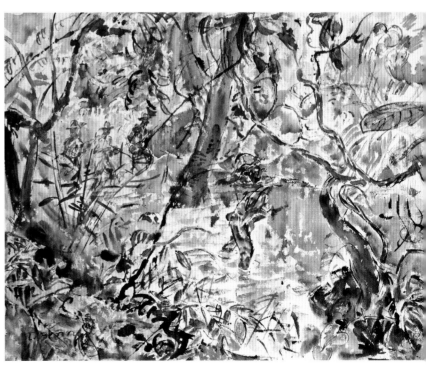

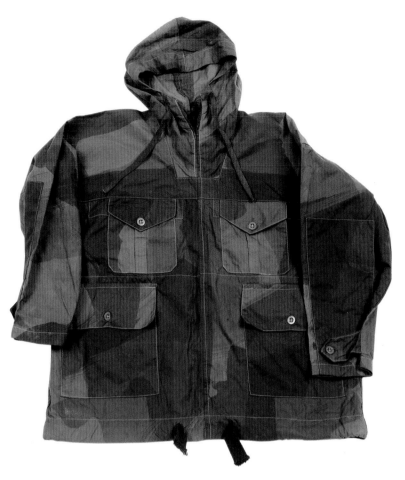

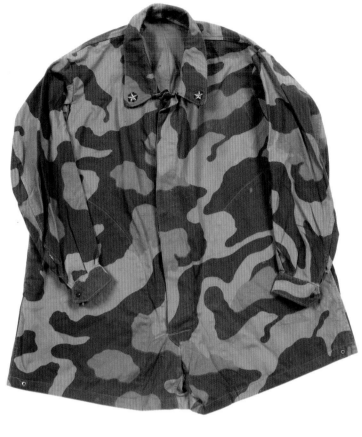

◢ **British windproofed camouflage jacket**. Part of a two-piece smock and trouser suit, this was intended to be worn as an over-suit. The pattern was unique to this suit and was initially popular with the Special Air Service and various commando units. In the latter stages of the Second World War, entire infantry units are known to have been issued with the suit during the winter of 1944–45 in Belgium.

◣ **Italian paratrooper's smock**. Camouflage clothing was frequently worn by specialist units throughout the Second World War and thus acquired an elite image.

two-piece utility uniform accompanied by a reversible camouflage helmet cover.

The pattern chosen for this camouflage combat dress was called 'frog-skin' and derived from experiments carried out by the US Army's Corps of Engineers in 1940. The winning design was chosen from one created by Norvell Gillespie, a horticulturist and gardening editor of *Better Homes and Gardens*. His inspiration came from the natural patterning on amphibians, consisting of abstract rounded shapes.

For combat purposes, the Marines' 'frog-skin' pattern was reproduced in two main colour combinations for reversible uniforms in the Pacific War zone – beach brown and jungle green. Some camouflage uniforms were issued in Europe to US soldiers during the Normandy invasion of 1944, but were rapidly withdrawn after other American soldiers confused their wearers with the German camouflage-clad Waffen-SS.

The importance of deriving inspiration from nature was underlined in the Smithsonian Institution War Background Studies booklet No.5 published in December 1942. Entitled *The Natural-History Background of Camouflage* and written by Herbert Friedmann, it paid full credit to the work of natural historians Abbott Thayer and Hugh Cott, who had thoroughly analysed camouflage in the animal kingdom. Friedmann recognized the

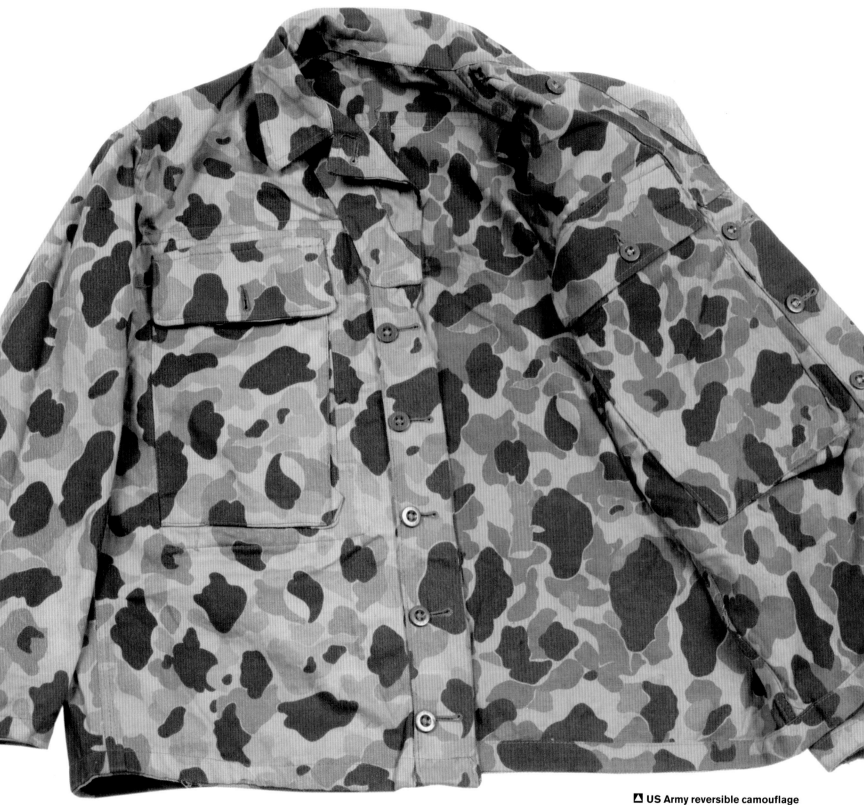

▲ **US Army reversible camouflage** issued in 1944. This pattern is often referred to as 'frog-skin'. On one side it is in light summer green colours, while the reverse shows darker tan autumnal shades.

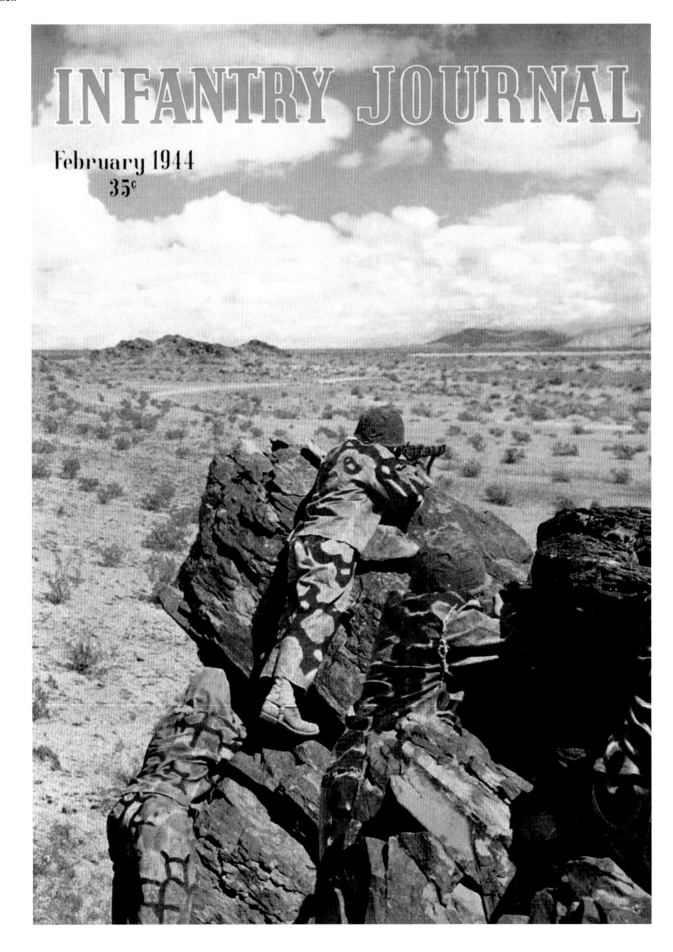

INFANTRY JOURNAL

February 1944
35¢

changes in modern warfare and declared 'it is probably no exaggeration to say that military camouflage has a greater and more vital importance now than it did in previous wars'. He presented his study as a quick primer in the understanding of natural camouflage for the interested military reader.

Experiments in different camouflage pattern uniforms continued in the United States throughout the war. The front cover of a 1944 issue of *Infantry Journal* showed trials for a black-striped disruptive pattern uniform in the Nevada desert, but the overall feedback on camouflage clothing worn in combat conditions was not good. The brown side of the 'frog-skin' pattern washed out to a bright pink and the two weights of fabric in the reversible uniform made it uncomfortably hot. Many US veterans believed a camouflage pattern made a moving soldier more obvious to the enemy than their usual green. This prejudice against camouflage combat dress contributed to its decline from 1943 onwards into the post-war period. Only Marine camouflaged helmet covers remained popular, and these stayed in use during the Korean and Vietnam Wars.

Francis S. Richardson, US Army Quartermaster consultant, produced a report on German camouflage combat clothing in 1945 and reinforced this prejudice. 'That the Germans made extensive use of camouflage fabrics is evident,' he wrote. 'Whether the results justified the effort is difficult to determine. Obviously white effects against the snow must have had some merit. The other types of effects are to be questioned. Talks with US Army combat officers would seem to bear out the fact that camouflage does not help if the object is in motion, be it a tank or a man. Objects which are stationary can be camouflaged and be very deceptive. In this regard several of these officers felt that the printed German shelter half [*Zeltbahn*] had merit, which would therefore suggest further study on this particular point.'

The effectiveness of disruptive pattern – its ability to break up forms and outlines, so making objects or individuals more difficult to detect, even against a shifting background – appears not to have been appreciated. The result was that camouflage combat dress hardly evolved in the US Army over the next twenty years.

The German army followed a different camouflage path. In 1931, it had adopted a camouflaged triangular tent sheet called a *Zeltbahn*, which could also double as a poncho. This followed on from the very first issue of camouflage material equipment to the Italian army in 1929 in the form of a tent with a disruptive pattern. The pattern chosen for the German army *Zeltbahn* was a composition of random green and brown angular shapes against a tan background with an overlay of green broken lines, looking like falling rain. It was called *Splitter* ('splinter') and derived from patterns applied to vehicles during the First World War.

◁ American experimental disruptive pattern camouflage combat clothing being tested in the Nevada desert, as illustrated on the cover of *Infantry Journal* magazine.

▽ German camouflage *Zeltbahn*, a triangular tent sheet that could also be used as a poncho. Issued in 1931, the *Zeltbahn* was the first step in the German army's introduction of camouflage clothing.

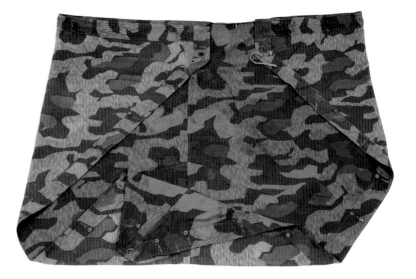

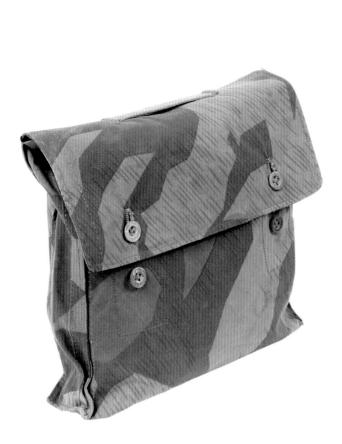

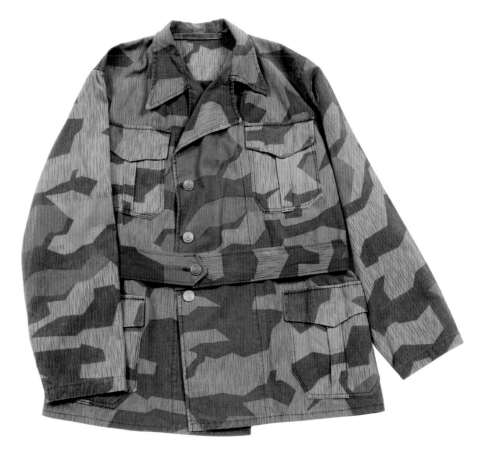

◢ **German *Splitter* pattern** on a bag. This was not regulation army issue, but has been made from an old camouflage jacket.

◥ **German *Splitter* pattern jacket.** This pattern was distinct from the tree-inspired designs worn by the Waffen-SS, the military arm of the Nazi Party (overleaf).

In 1941, the *Splitter* pattern was used on a jump smock worn by paratroopers during the invasion of Crete. In 1943, the German army introduced a variant of *Splitter* in which the sharp edges of the angular shapes were softened to create a blurred pattern called *Sumpfmuster* or 'marsh pattern'. A shortage of high quality cotton duck material during the war meant that production of camouflage clothing was limited and it remained the badge of elite assault soldiers.

Splitter pattern and its variants were very different from the camouflage patterns worn by the Nazi Party's elite Waffen-SS fighting units. The Waffen-SS had already devised its own distinctive forest-inspired camouflage prints before the start of the war (overleaf), and continued to experiment with different patterns throughout the war. Among these, a pattern evolved out of the oak-leaf form called *Erbsenmuster* or 'pea pattern', consisting of round splodges in shades of black, green, and dark and light brown. Finally, in 1945, appeared *Leibermuster* – a striking pattern seemingly designed for winter urban fighting, featuring ragged black stripes over dark green and reddish brown splodges against a light green background. It contained a light-absorbing dye to counter detection by infra-red night sights. It was not widely issued and only a handful of uniforms survive.

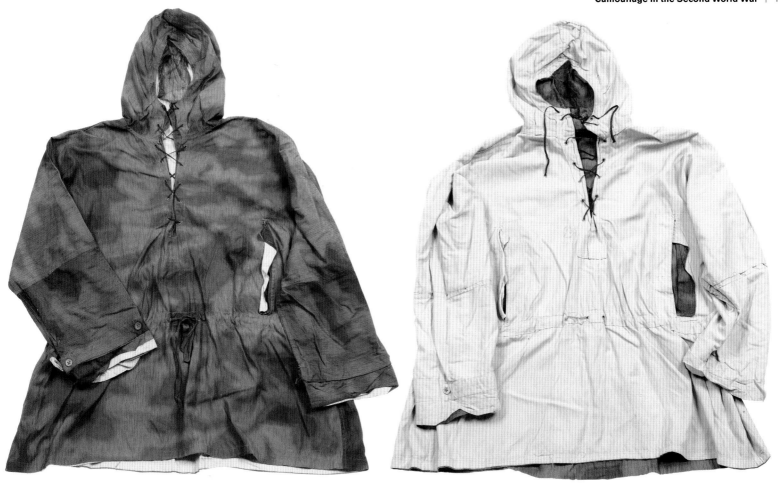

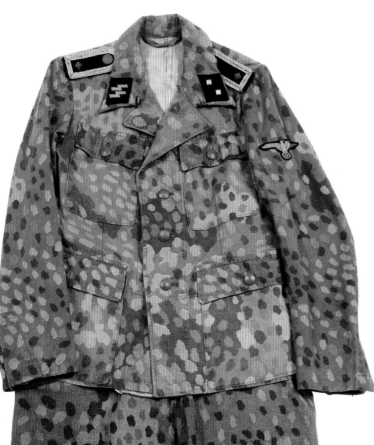

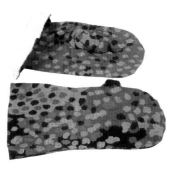

▲ **German *Sumpfmuster* smock, reversible to white** (both sides shown). *Sumpfmuster* was a blurred form of the *Splitter* pattern.

◀▼ **German Waffen-SS combat jacket, trousers and mittens** in so-called *Erbsenmuster* or 'pea pattern', introduced in 1944.

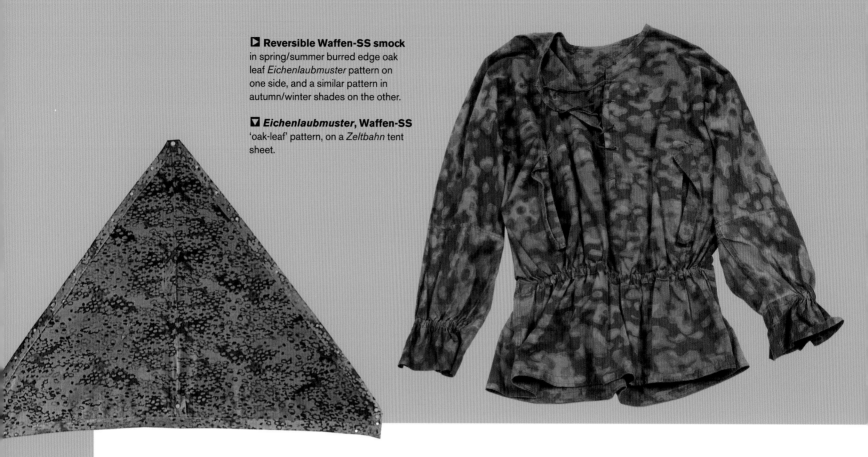

▶ **Reversible Waffen-SS smock**
in spring/summer burred edge oak
leaf *Eichenlaubmuster* pattern on
one side, and a similar pattern in
autumn/winter shades on the other.

▼ *Eichenlaubmuster*, **Waffen-SS**
'oak-leaf' pattern, on a *Zeltbahn* tent
sheet.

Patterns of the Forest

The very first mass-produced camouflage uniforms
were invented in Germany in the 1930s. Unlike
the patterns of the First World War, which were
mainly geometric and utilitarian in origin, these first
manufactured textile camouflage patterns were
inspired by the forest.

Two thousand years before the First World War,
German warriors ambushed a Roman army in the
Teutoburgian forest and wiped it out, stopping
dead any further Roman conquest of Germany.
Hitler commissioned a tapestry for his headquarters
commemorating this ancient victory. The German
forest also produced expert hunters and rifle-
armed, green-jacketed elite warriors.

With such reverence for their forest background,
it is little surprise that the most fanatical of all
German military groups, the Waffen-SS, should
have sought inspiration in tree forms when
designing a camouflage uniform. The Waffen-SS
was the military arm of the Nazi Party. SS Major
Wim Brandt, a doctor of engineering and

commander of reconnaissance, began the search
for a new form of camouflage pattern. He found it
in the work of Munich-based Professor Otto Schick.

A later American report on the process said that
Schick 'had made a study of the effect of sunlight
through trees both in the summer when they were
in full leaf and in the autumn when all vegetation
was dried and brown. In this manner he achieved
his color combinations and some of the fabrics
produced had the green combination on one side
and the brown on the other.'

The result of Schick's research were three main
forms of tree pattern. These were the 'plane tree'
or *Platanenmuster*, the 'palm tree' or *Palmenmuster*,
and the 'oak leaf' or *Eichenlaubmuster*. We do not
know the original names of these patterns; these
titles were applied by collectors after the war.

The *Platanenmuster* appears to be among
the earliest of Schick's patterns and is closest
in appearance to flaking plane tree bark. The
Palmenmuster is the least abstract of all the

patterns, incorporating drawings of leaves, but
the pattern is in fact not based on the palm tree.
Instead, it shows bunches of long feather-like
leaves, possibly ash, alongside spots and furry
blobs representing seed pods or fruits. The most
widely used of the early Waffen-SS patterns
was the *Eichenlaubmuster*. This looked most like
clusters of lobed oak leaves and was produced
in green and brown versions.

In 1937, the prototype camouflage patterns of
Schick and Brandt were tested in field manoeuvres
and were estimated to reduce casualties by
15 per cent. The following year, a patent was
awarded by the Reich Patent Office for the forest
patterns on a reversible spring green/autumn
brown camouflage helmet cover, pullover smock,
and sniper face-mask. The patent meant that the
German army could not copy the patterns and
these tree motifs became the distinctive
camouflage of the Waffen-SS.

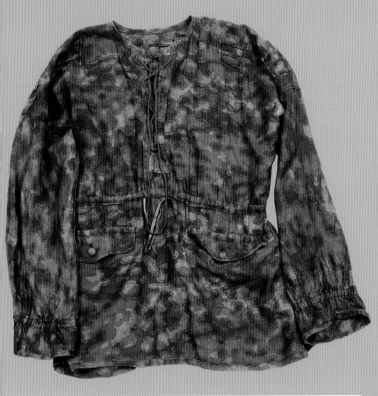

◀ **Waffen-SS smock** in autumn/winter burred edge oak leaf *Eichenlaubmuster* pattern. Strips of cloth are fixed in threes to the upper chest, shoulders and neck to allow foliage to be attached for greater personal concealment.

▶ **German recruiting poster** for the Waffen-SS in occupied Belgium. This features a soldier wearing the distinctive Waffen-SS tree-derived camouflage pattern as a helmet cover.

▼ **Waffen-SS smock** in *Palmenmuster* pattern, which features elements that resemble ash leaves and seed pods.

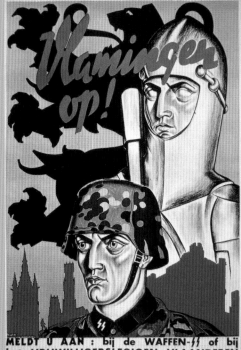

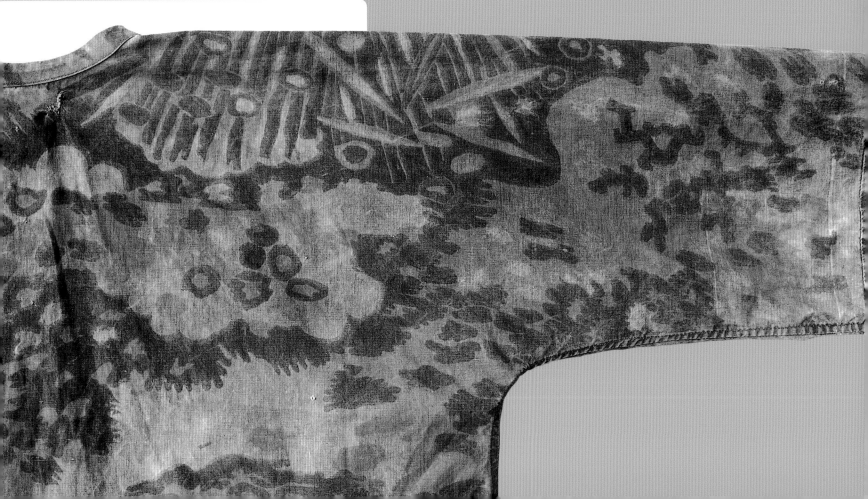

Painting Tanks and Ships

Camouflage began in the First World War as a method of protecting artillery and vehicles and this continued into the Second World War. The French, as the originators of painted camouflage, had all their tanks covered in a variety of distinct patterns, including: simple olive green with chocolate brown blotches; horizontal wavy green and brown lines edged with darker brown outlines; vertical green and sand wavy lines with dark brown outlines. Despite their pioneering work in camouflage combat dress, the Germans seemed reluctant to follow the French example and their tanks during the early *Blitzkrieg* period were mainly painted a dark grey, known as *Panzergrau*.

Desert warfare in North Africa meant that tanks were easily exposed against the low horizons and so every army was forced to adopt camouflage patterns. The British were the most distinctive,

◪ **Experimental sketches of tank camouflage schemes** devised at the British Camouflage Development and Training Centre. The disruptive patterns of black and khaki green blocks separated by a white line were designed to make the tank more difficult for the enemy to target accurately.

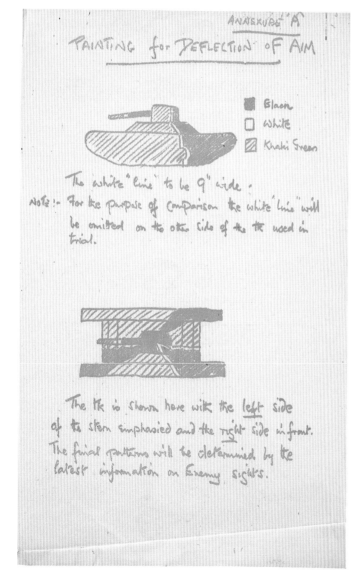

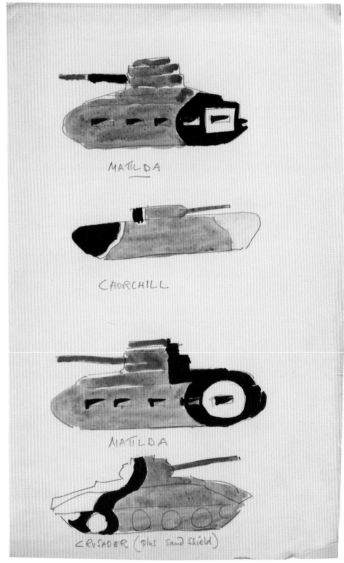

with horizontal bands of sand, dark brown and sky blue painted on their tanks, more in the spirit of Dazzle camouflage, using the sky colour to completely disrupt the vehicle profile. Other nations, including Germany, used a variety of sand shades.

The British tested different camouflage schemes throughout the war. Sketches of patterns devised for Matilda and Churchill tanks survive in the papers of Major Denys Pavitt of the Camouflage Development and Training Centre. Their stated intention was to deflect the aim of enemy sights, much like Dazzle painting on ships in the First World War. These schemes consisted of ragged areas of black and khaki green paint separated by a white line some 9 inches (23 cm) wide, thus giving the illusion of breaking the tank in half.

On the Eastern Front from 1941 onwards, the Germans became more inventive with their tank camouflage. Many tanks intended

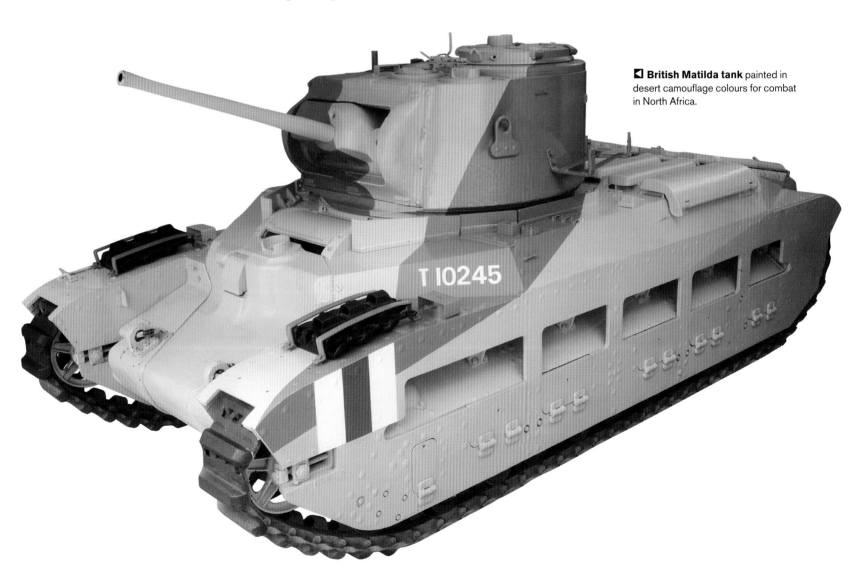

British Matilda tank painted in desert camouflage colours for combat in North Africa.

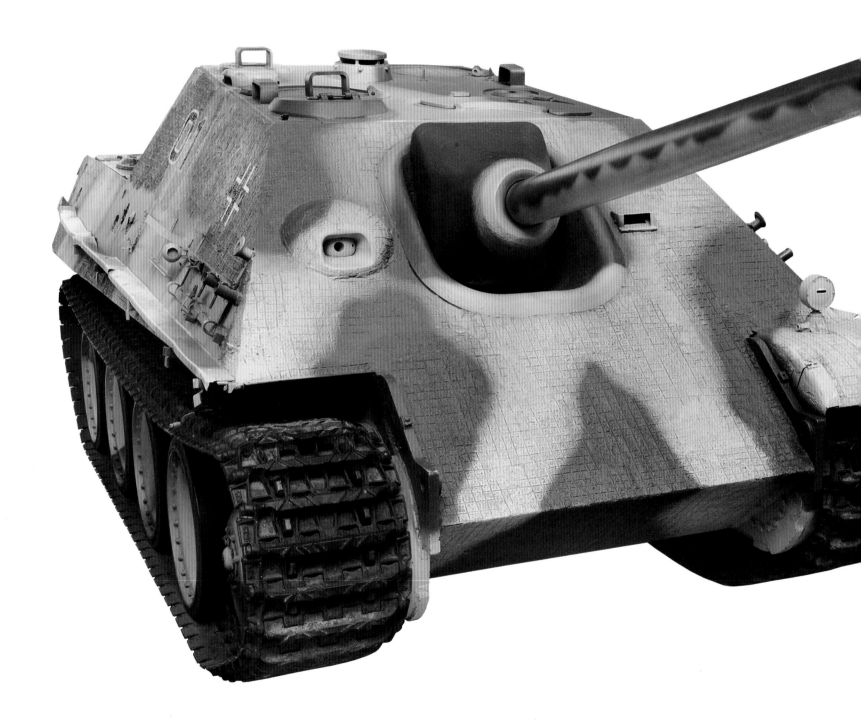

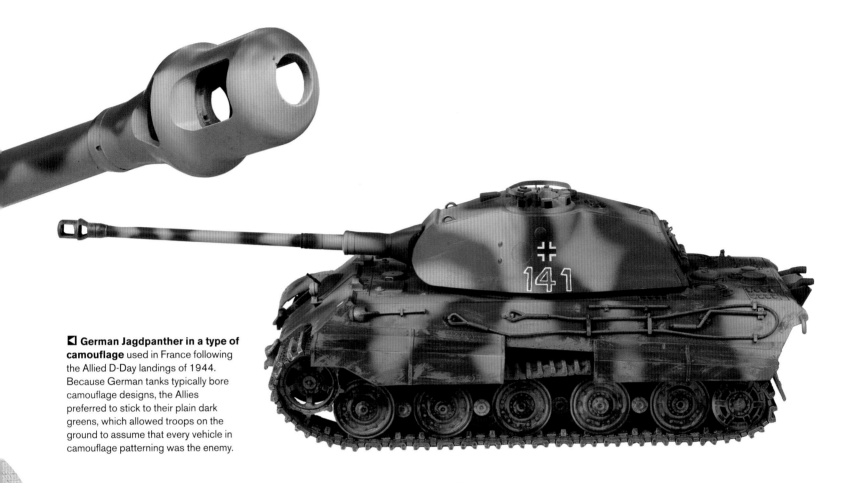

◀ **German Jagdpanther in a type of camouflage** used in France following the Allied D-Day landings of 1944. Because German tanks typically bore camouflage designs, the Allies preferred to stick to their plain dark greens, which allowed troops on the ground to assume that every vehicle in camouflage patterning was the enemy.

▲ **Model of camouflaged German Tiger II.** The 'King Tiger' was introduced in the autumn of 1944, during the Allied advance towards Germany, by which time German tanks were painted in an array of striking camouflage patterns.

for North Africa were redirected to Russia where their sand-coloured finish worked well against the dusty steppes. Individual tank crews were encouraged to paint their own camouflage patterns on their vehicles and were supplied with pots of paint and spray equipment. Sometimes great care was taken, creating striped or spotted schemes, but other times soldiers would just throw pots of paint against the sides of their vehicles.

During the winter, German crews applied whitewash to lessen tanks' visibility, not making them completely white, but simply smearing the whitewash on so that it merged with the snow and mud. In the spring, it could be easily removed. Soviet tanks were generally dark green, but whitewash was also used to lessen their visibility and help them merge with the snowy landscape.

In 1944 in northern Europe, following the D-Day invasion, Allied troops came up against the most brightly camouflaged German tanks of all. Since February 1943, German tanks had been painted in a base colour of dark yellow rather than grey. Panzer units were also issued with two more colours, drab olive and red-brown, which could be applied over the yellow base in disruptive patterns. There were tanks painted in stripes, splinter and lozenge schemes, and even in a storm of spots known as ambush camouflage because it worked well against the dappled shade of leaves. The Allies kept mainly to dark greens for their own tanks, largely because it became easy to assume everything in camouflage was the enemy and so could be fired on.

After the spectacle of Dazzle ships in the First World War, there had been a return to more orthodox colouring. At the outset of the Second World War, grey predominated in the British Navy and there were no systematic plans for camouflaging warships. Martin Chisolm, a naval officer aboad H.M.S. *Duke of York*, recalled how at the beginning of the conflict 'the fancies of individual command-ing officers rather than the dictates of scientific observation often decided how particular groups of warships should be painted in the early days.'

This changed when the British Naval Research Laboratory at Teddington established a group of artists and scientists at the local art gallery in Leamington Spa. Led by Commander James Yunge-Bateman, their task was to revisit the work of Norman Wilkinson and devise new forms of camouflage. They chose two paths. One was to create colour schemes that would enable a ship to blend into particular environments. This worked especially well when choosing colours for landing craft at D-Day, when the exact geography of the seascape was known well.

When there could be no attempt to hide from the enemy, then camouflage had to deceive the eye, making a ship a more difficult target for the enemy. This meant Dazzle-style disruptive pattern, and many new schemes were designed and tested on models floating in tanks viewed under different lights and against differ-ent backgrounds. Specially devised viewing machines would recreate the effects of hazy conditions at sea. Naval officer James Chisholm observed that this was an area that particularly suited the talents of artists recruited to the naval laboratory.

'Perhaps a modern abstract artist like Picasso,' he said, 'would be the most helpful of all working on camouflage schemes, for he would have at his command a deep knowledge of abstract design which could find ready scope.'

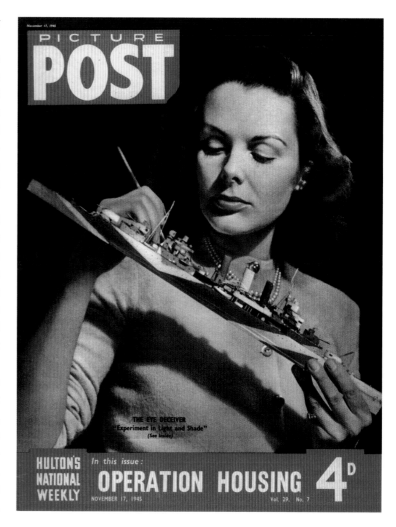

◩ **Cover of *Picture Post* in November 1945,** finally revealing the wartime work of British naval *camoufleurs* in designing patterns to disguise ships. As in the First World War, these were first developed and tested on models before being scaled up to full size.

◩ ***Donning their Battledress; Liners and Cargo Vessels being Camouflaged,*** watercolour by Thomas Halliday, 1947. The British and US navies used Dazzle-style camouflage on some of their vessels as a protection against against the perils of German U-Boats during the Second World War.

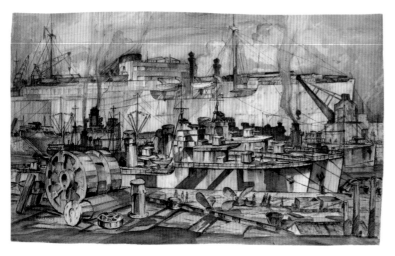

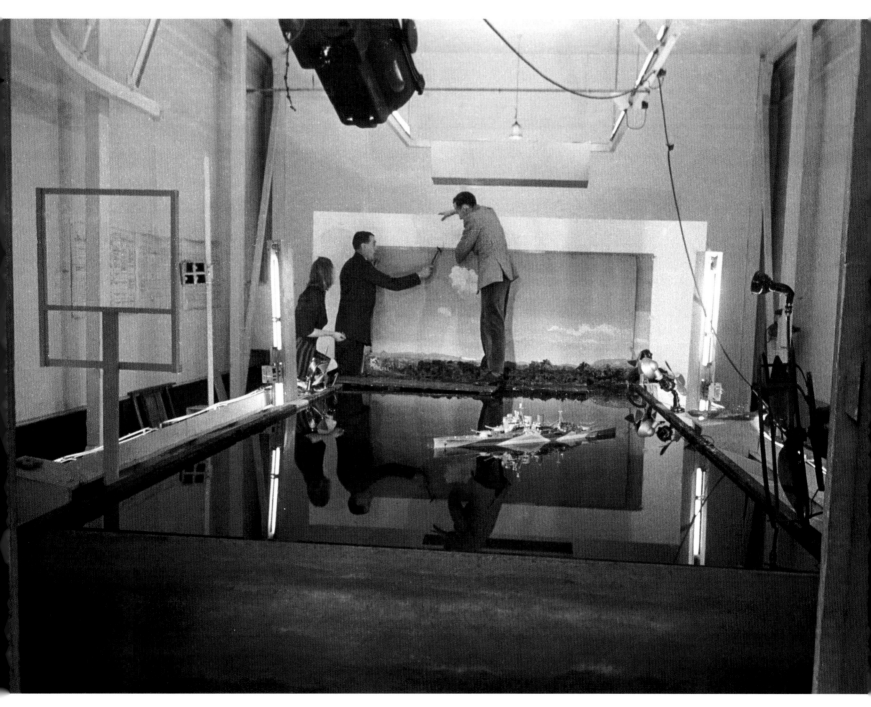

▲ **Staff of the British Naval Research Laboratory** at Leamington Spa test the effectiveness of camouflage schemes on painted models viewed against various backgrounds.

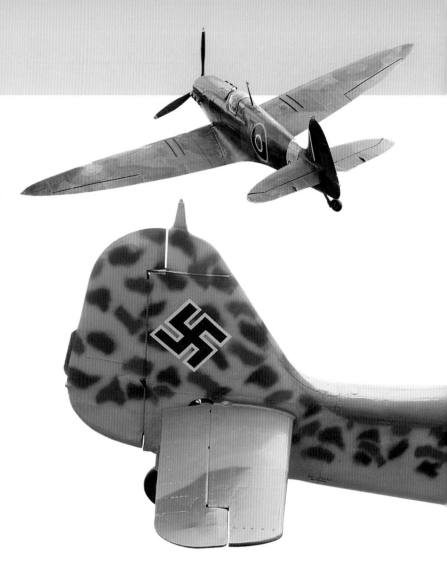

Aircraft Camouflage

The British RAF deployed disruptive pattern camouflage throughout the war on their fighter planes, but they were sensitive to the changing demands of battle. In summer 1941, they altered their camouflage to confront a switch in tactics by the *Luftwaffe*. German fighter planes were flying at higher altitudes, at which British pilots reported their own dark green, dark brown and sky blue scheme appeared conspicuously dark. They were losing pilots as a result. After trials by the Air Fighting Development Unit at Duxford, the dark brown was replaced by 'Ocean Grey'; this was matched by a so-called 'Sea Grey' on the underside, replacing the sky blue.

The Germans went through a similar process as they fought for survival against high-performing Allied fighter planes. Dark green splinter patterns were changed for more muted stippled and mottled schemes, providing improved high-altitude concealment. The Americans favoured 'Dark Olive Drab' on the upper surfaces and fuselage sides of their aircraft, with a 'Neutral Grey' on the undersides. The US Navy did experiment with striking disruptive patterns on their torpedo planes, but the results were negative. Allied air superiority towards the end of the war meant that camouflage became less important and American pilots flew in unpainted silver aircraft straight from the factory.

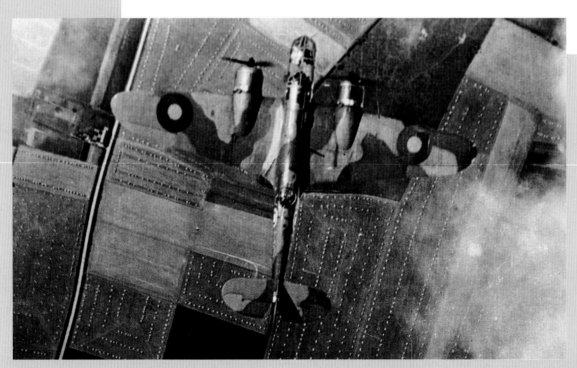

◀ **Bristol Blenheim Mark IV** in flight over countryside, its camouflage scheme echoing the light and dark tones of the fields beneath it.

▶ **Model of British Hawker Hurricane Mark I** in typical Allied camouflage pattern.

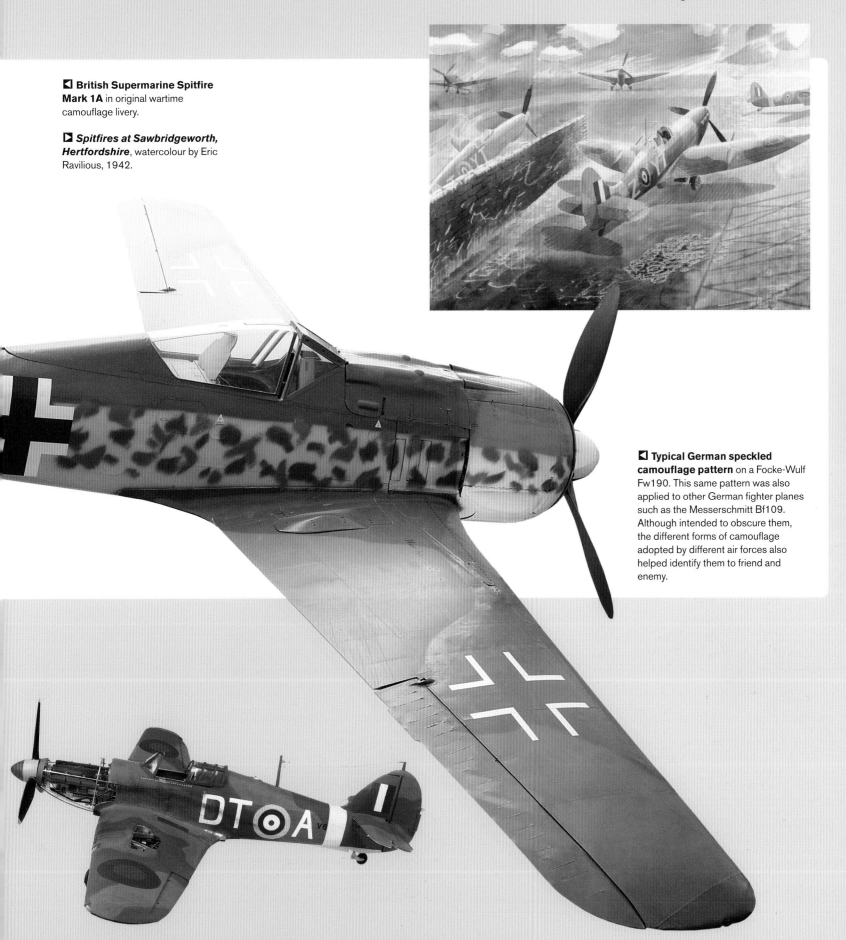

◀ **British Supermarine Spitfire Mark 1A** in original wartime camouflage livery.

▶ *Spitfires at Sawbridgeworth, Hertfordshire*, watercolour by Eric Ravilious, 1942.

◀ **Typical German speckled camouflage pattern** on a Focke-Wulf Fw190. This same pattern was also applied to other German fighter planes such as the Messerschmitt Bf109. Although intended to obscure them, the different forms of camouflage adopted by different air forces also helped identify them to friend and enemy.

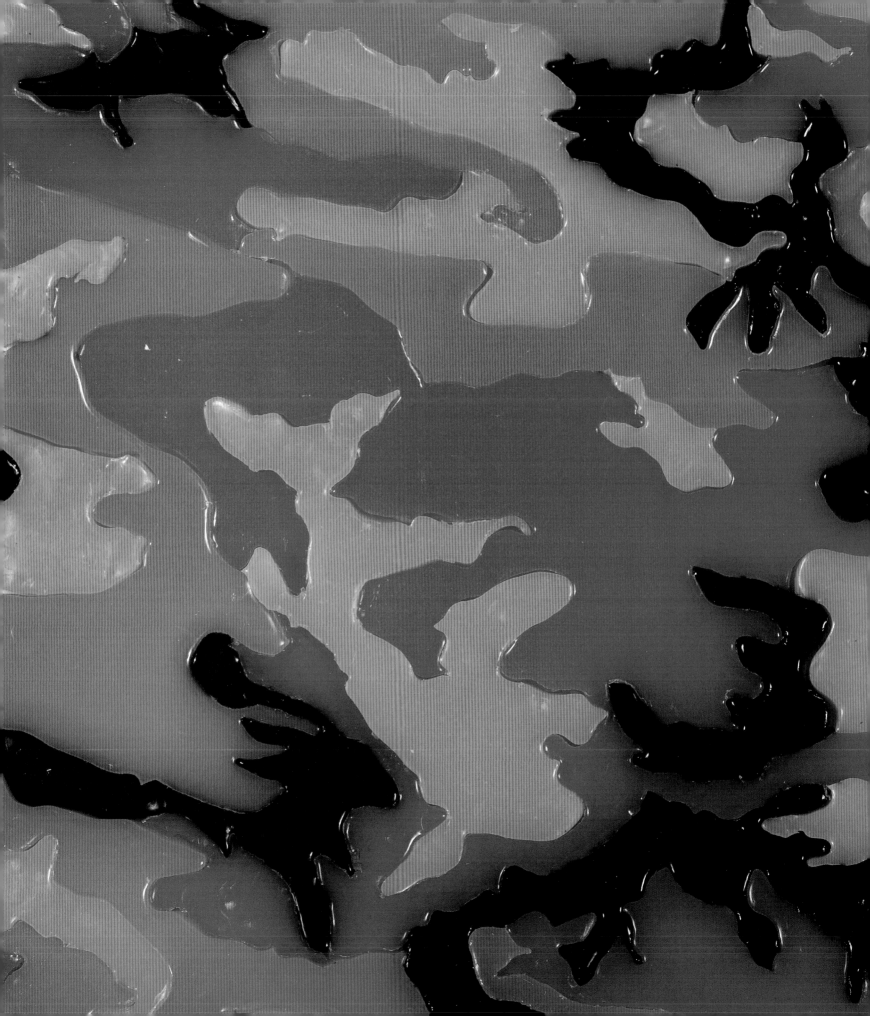

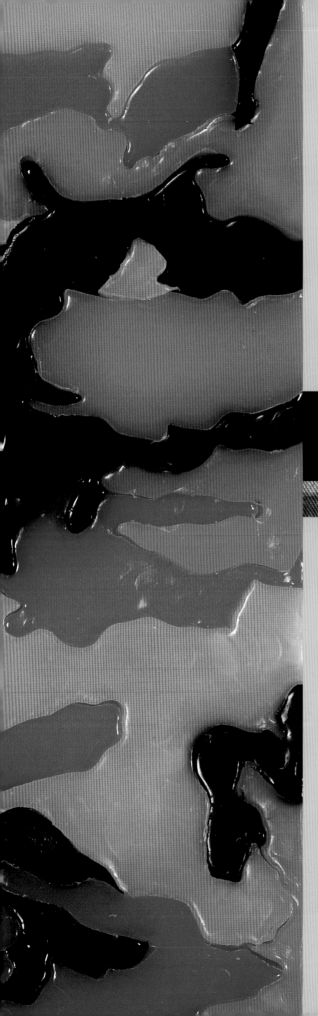

Camo Triumphant
Camouflage in War and Peace since 1945

The conflicts of the Cold War period again proved the military value of camouflage. But as disruptive pattern became virtually synonymous with combat clothing, so it also acquired a far wider range of associations. Worn by anti-war protesters; appropriated by hip hop groups; explored by artists and designers; appearing in street fashion and on the catwalk – camouflage became the universal style icon that we know today.

Camo Triumphant
Camouflage in War and Peace since 1945

In the 21st century, camouflage is everywhere: not just on high fashion and street fashion but everything from children's pyjamas and duvet covers, to milkshake cups, skateboards, sticky tape, pencils, erasers, slippers and ties. It is one of the most popular forms of decoration on the planet. Its wide appeal to the civilian world is matched by its dominance in military life. Most armies have their own distinct camouflage battledress – in many cases with several different patterns for different areas of operation. But this triumphant outcome was by no means inevitable. Indeed, it looked for some years as though earlier wartime experiments in combat camouflage might be abandoned in a Cold War world of confrontation between nuclear superpowers.

Camouflage in Doubt

In Britain in 1960, there was a high-level military dispute over an item of clothing. This heated debate was about the Denison Smock – the British Army's first major venture into camouflage battledress which had been first issued to the Parachute Regiment in 1941 (see page 129). Should it stay or should it go?

In 1957–58, a worldwide trial took place of a new British combat suit and one of the units taking part in the tests came from the Parachute Regiment. The combat clothing proved successful and it was recommended that it be issued throughout the British Army, including the Paras, in 1961. This new combat clothing did not carry a disruptive camouflage pattern, and it was noted at the time that further tests would need to be done before this was applied. In the meantime, the new combat outfit was to replace the camouflaged Denison Smock, worn since the Second World War. This was the recommendation of the Quartermaster General (QMG), the office responsible for the supply of military equipment.

Once this news reached the Paras, they were not so sure. Brigadier Napier Crookenden, commander of the 16th Parachute Brigade Group, wrote a letter to the Under-Secretary of State at the War Office, in August 1960, expressing the concerns of his soldiers. 'The airborne smock has been worn since 1940,' he wrote, 'and has been a distinctive feature of airborne forces since that year. It has since been copied and adopted by the SAS, Royal Marines, Amphibious Observation Regiment RA and other special forces.' Crookenden then listed the practical virtues of the Denison Smock, noting 'it looks serviceable and warlike and is popular with its wearers.'

His emphasis on the camouflage smock's distinctiveness and popularity with soldiers is worth noting. Throughout the history of military costume, it has frequently been not only the practical function of an item of combat clothing that endears it to soldiers, but also its impressive and warlike appearance – and camouflage patterning very much shares that appeal.

▶ A US military surplus M65 Woodland camouflage jacket
bearing imagery from Stanley Kubrick's film *2001: A Space Odyssey*, created by British designer Hardy Blechman for his Maharishi fashion label's spring/summer 2004 collection.

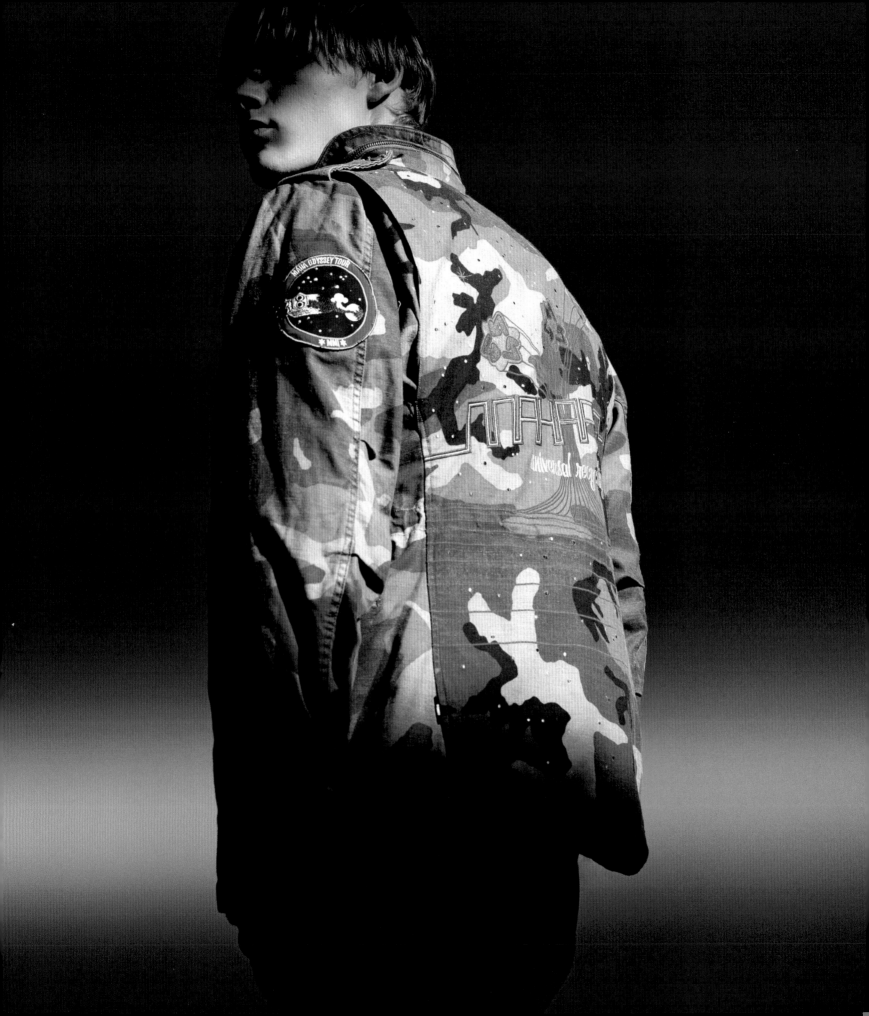

'We want to keep our airborne smock,' concluded the Brigade commander, 'because it is practical, distinctive and honoured by long usage. The Highland regiment are provided with a much less practical and far more expensive garment, in which to parade [the Highland kilt]. Let us go on fighting and training in our Airborne Smock.'

Crookenden's letter caused a stir among senior figures of the military establishment. The Vice Quartermaster General considered it 'a rather tricky matter' and admitted that 'morale counts for the hell of a lot.' Other senior officers disagreed. 'Nor can I put it [the Denison Smock] in the same class as the kilt,' said one, 'which is a *national* garment of many centuries standing. It would be almost as logical to ask that Riflemen should wear the same uniform that they retreated from Corunna in [the green uniform of 1809], as to retain the smock.'

As this controversy raged, an officer of the Quartermaster General visited the United States to discuss their research into the effectiveness of camouflage combat clothing. The official US Army view in 1961 was that disruptive pattern on clothing had no real advantage over a single colour that blended with the natural background. At a later NATO meeting, another office of the QMG spoke to their German allies who had retained Disruptive Pattern clothing since the end of the war, but were told that they too had decided to revert to a single colour for their combat uniforms. This global lack of interest in uniform camouflage further marginalized those arguing for the survival of the Denison Smock in the British Army.

The final nail in its coffin came when the QMG explained that they had always found it hard to find a commercial firm willing to take on the task of printing camouflage fabric for the Denison Smock. This problem had also prevented its wider use in the rest of the British Army.

'This difficulty frequently causes delay in obtaining smocks,' reported the Assistant QMG in April 1961, 'and production is held up until the printing process can be undertaken during a gap in normal production. If a decision was made that the combat clothing should be camouflaged then the production problem would be a serious one. It would be extremely difficult, if not impossible, to find a firm willing to undertake this work on a large scale.'

So, for this practical reason, camouflage combat dress was not adopted into the British Army for the best part of another decade, and the fate of the Denison Smock was sealed. Despite being recognized as a vital part of the tradition of the Parachute Regiment, it was replaced by a new plain suit, though it was retained for a few further years for use in tropical zones.

This early Cold War disinterest in disruptive pattern camouflage could be found in other branches of the military service too. The

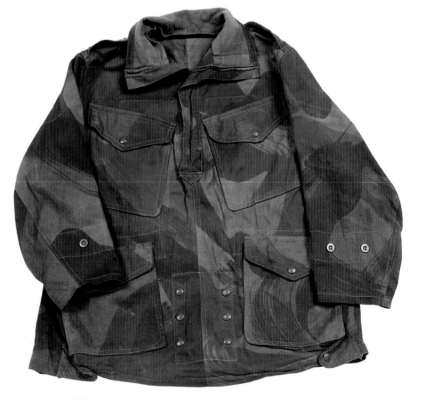

◥ **British Denison Smock**. By 1960, this camouflaged combat jacket had become a favourite item of the Parachute Regiment and a government threat to discontinue it provoked a protest from the regimental commander. Even so, it was replaced by a plain-coloured suit in 1961, as military authorities across the West turned their backs on camouflage combat gear in the post-war years.

most striking example of this was in the US Air Force. Since 1944 their new jet aircraft had been dispatched directly from the factory to the frontline in brilliant, naked, silver metal. They had no need to daub their ultra-fast fighter-bombers in camouflage colours. Overwhelming air superiority made such disguise redundant.

All this military indifference to camouflage changed towards the end of the 1960s. The reason for this – Vietnam.

New Heraldry

One major difference between the two world wars and the conflicts of the Cold War era was that after 1945, although many regular soldiers were still conscripted, military establishments were staffed mainly by professional career warriors. In the two world wars, amateurs had flooded in. Their presence goes some way to explaining the prevalence of colourful camouflage patterning. Many amateur soldiers in camouflage units were artists who brought their aesthetic interests with them. In the immediate post-war era, there was little artistry to military camouflage.

The development of camouflage was left to military scientists in both Britain and the United States. In the United Kingdom, a Camouflage Laboratory was set up in Didcot, Berkshire, as part of the Directorate of Stores and Clothing Development. In 1960, it tested the effectiveness of khaki and green as camouflage colours in tropical regions – but there was no reference whatsoever to disruptive patterning, whose attributes were not considered sufficiently scientific.

Many senior military figures simply didn't like camouflage. One RAF Air Marshal expressed strong feelings about the appearance of his fighter aircraft: 'Some of our aircraft, in my opinion, look a mess,' he wrote in April 1967, 'over-painted with fussy schemes which fight ineffectually against enough printed instructions on their skins to provide a morning's reading.... But if it is therefore essential that we paint aircraft I suggest that we should be practical, simple, and reasonably aesthetic.' This meant a monochrome finish.

The United States Air Force only considered painting its silver-skinned jet fighters when it was noticed that aircraft sitting on runways in Southeast Asia were deteriorating alarmingly fast. In 1966, a seventy-page report on the Phantom revealed that the effect of a humid saline atmosphere on unprotected aluminium alloy was to nearly eat it through. Reports on other aircraft showed a similarly high level of corrosion. Having decided to paint their aircraft, the Americans turned to their British comrades for advice on suitable camouflage colours.

The conflict in Vietnam also had a tremendous impact on the wearing of camouflaged patterned uniforms by American soldiers. Most troops entering the conflict in 1965 looked little different

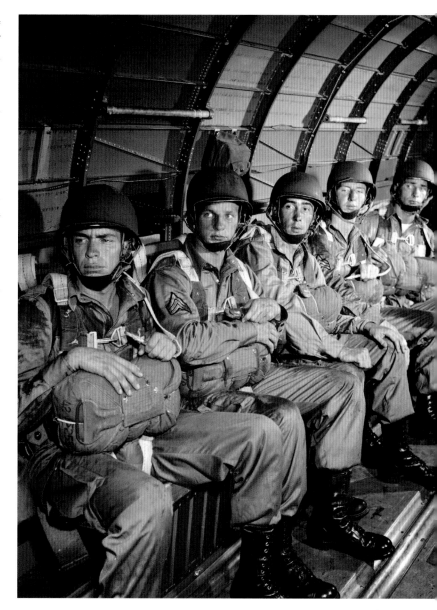

◤ **US Army Airborne paratroopers** in a C-47 transport aircraft. By the late 1950s, camouflage clothing had fallen out of favour in the US Army, whose authorities disputed the effectiveness of disruptive pattern prints and preferred single colour combat dress.

⬇ **Vietnamese soldiers using local
foliage** for camouflage cover.
Photograph by Tim Page.

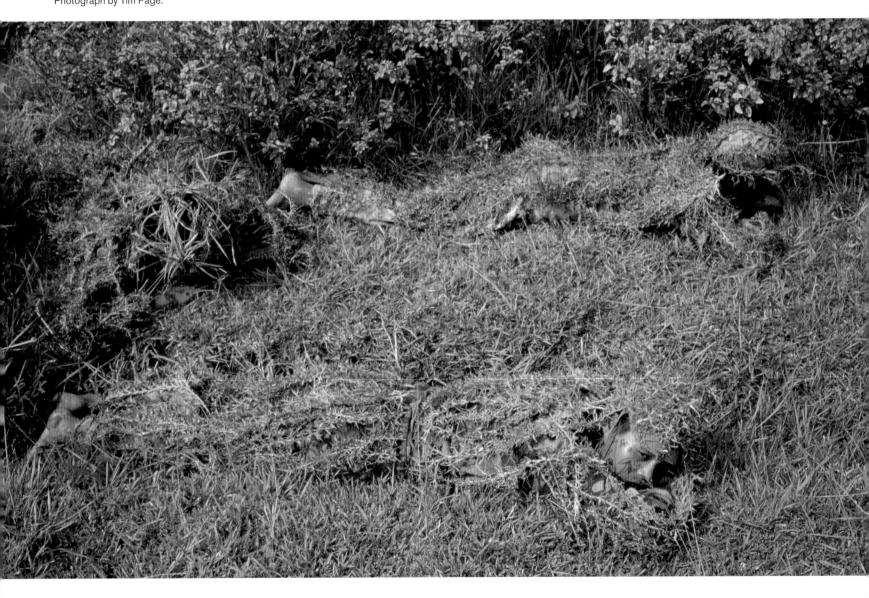

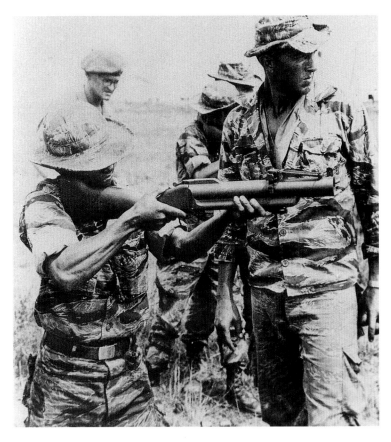

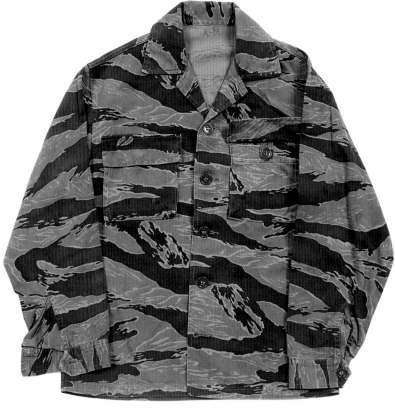

from those that fought in the Second World War. The only remnant of camouflage was a 'leaves and twigs' helmet cover that super-seded the 'frog-skin' pattern helmet cover worn by the US Marines. Otherwise, they wore monochrome uniforms. However, if the first US military advisors to South Vietnam could not draw upon official army camouflage clothing, they could – and did – use CIA funds to buy 'duck hunter' camouflage from civilian shops back in the US, such as Sears Roebuck.

As the conflict expanded, the need for camouflage clothing became clear and US military advisors turned to their South Vietnamese comrades for inspiration. The Vietnamese Marine Corps, an elite branch of the Republic of Vietnam army, had been wearing their own distinctive 'tiger-stripe' pattern since 1959. This consisted of black horizontal stripes printed over a light and dark green background. This, in turn, may have been derived from the 'lizard' pattern worn by French paratroopers serving in Indo-China in 1953.

This attractive, aggressive pattern soon gained tremendous prestige among US soldiers and was worn by reconnaissance and Special Forces units. American funding allowed it to be produced on a large scale in factories in Japan, Thailand, Taiwan and Korea. It even became fashionable to wear tiger-stripe on vacation in the form of swimming trunks.

▼ Tiger-stripe camouflage worn by a US military advisor and a South Vietnamese member of the Civilian Irregular Defense Group during the war in Vietnam.

◣ Shirt in tiger-stripe camouflage which is believed to have been first worn by the Vietnamese Marine Corps from 1959. Adopted by individual US Special Forces advisors during the earlier stages of the Vietnam Conflict, the pattern was subsequently taken up by other elite formations, including those of Australia and New Zealand. In the mid-1960s the South Vietnamese adopted tiger-stripe uniforms for their own Ranger Battalions.

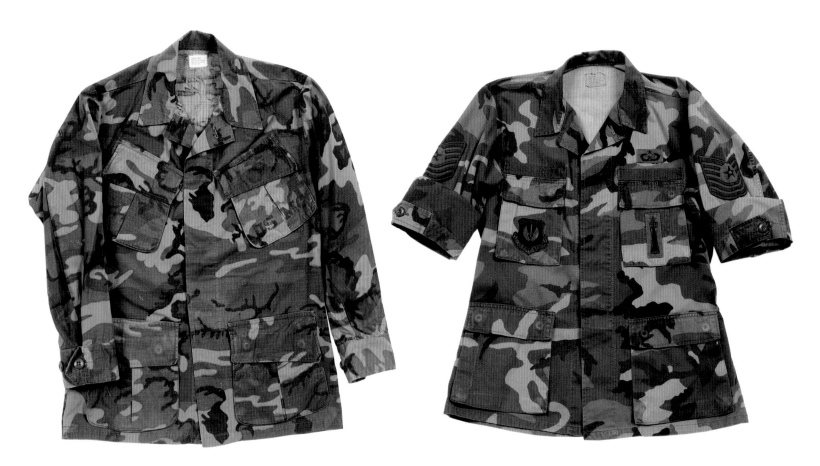

◢ Woodland variant camouflage pattern on a US Marine Corps jacket. This pattern was adopted by the Marine Corps in 1968.

◢ M81 Woodland camouflage pattern on a US Air Force jacket.

Seeing its success both practically and for morale, US military opinion swung behind the production of camouflage and an early form of the classic US 'Woodland' leaf-style pattern was released from 1967. At first this was issued to elite units, but then to the rest of the army, so that by the end of the Vietnam War, American troops wearing camouflage combat dress had become the norm. This represented a tremendous revolution in the acceptance of disruptive patterned military clothing and set the tone for the rest of the world's military forces. Now, everyone wanted to wear camouflage combat dress – even the British.

By the early 1970s, Britain was looking to the United States for advances in camouflage clothing. The British Army had finally adopted its own distinctive disruptive pattern material (DPM), consisting of a green, brown and a black brush-stroke motif, which, ironically, was derived from that of the discontinued Denison Smock. US pattern ideas came from the Natick Research, Development and Engineering Center. Their new – now iconic – 'chocolate-chip' desert pattern was tested in 1973 against British DPM by the Stores and Clothing Research and Development Establishment in Colchester, Essex. Which was best?

The two patterns were viewed with the naked eye against foliage backgrounds and also through infra-red binoculars and were photographed. 'On the monochrome and infra-red photo-

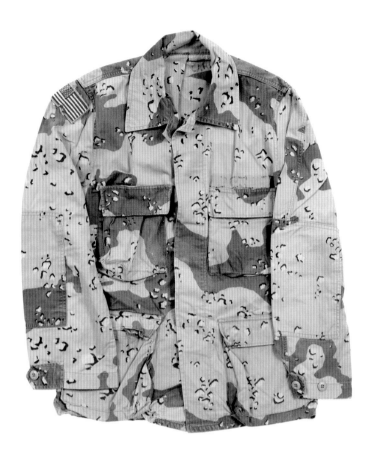

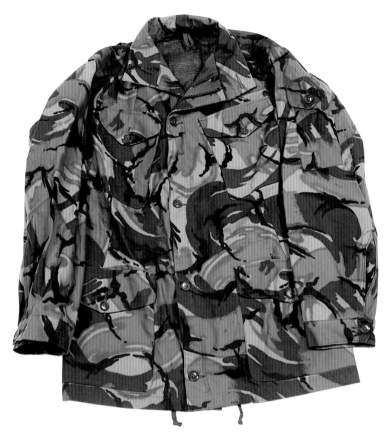

graphs,' concluded the report, 'the American jacket was much more conspicuous than the British. Also, it was easier to detect with the naked eye up to distances of about 150 metres. Seen though infra-red binoculars, however, there was not a great deal of difference between the infra-red performance of the two jackets, although at the longer distances the British jacket appeared slightly superior.'

In fact, it was a good result for the desert pattern as the comparison was unfair: unlike British DPM, it was not designed for the temperate-zone setting in which the tests were conducted. A closer result was obtained when an experimental US temperate-zone jacket was tested – this was a dark chequered pattern primarily intended to thwart night-time observational devices. 'The camouflaging properties of the two jackets were good,' said the report. 'Mostly they resembled each other very closely in appearance.'

It is interesting to note the early date of development of the chocolate-chip desert pattern, which only became widely known during the Gulf War of 1991, some twenty years later. Curiously, it was soon after dropped from the army as the chocolate-chip motif proved unpopular among its troops, who felt it didn't look military enough. The replacement desert pattern (see page 156) is a simpler design which, according to the official US line, has an improved 'psychological effect and is a morale booster'.

◪ **US chocolate-chip desert warfare camouflage**. First developed in the early 1970s, this iconic pattern became widely recognized during the Gulf War of 1991, but was shortly afterwards dropped by the US Army.

◪ **British DPM combat jacket**, 1968 pattern. This classic 'brush-stroke' pattern was derived from that used on the Denison Smock first issued during the Second World War and discontinued in 1961.

Following the second US-led conflict with Iraq in 2003, the left-over stock of chocolate-chip desert uniforms was distributed to members of the newly re-created Iraqi army – soldiers intended to take over security responsibilities from coalition forces. This was an excellent example of camouflage combat uniforms being used not just to hide soldiers but also to identify them to each other.

Camouflage patterning has become the new heraldry of the 21st century. British DPM is as readily recognized by friend and foe as British scarlet used to be in the 19th century.

A similar process occurred in camouflage uniform development elsewhere in the world through the last phase of the Cold War. The soldiers of US client states wore Woodland-style patterns, while Eastern Bloc allies of the Soviet Union copied their jigsaw and small leaf patterns. Nationalism, however, also raised its head and some states devised their own distinct patterns to reinforce

◹ **A US soldier (right) in new desert pattern camouflage** on patrol with an Iraqi soldier wearing old US chocolate-chip desert camouflage. These patterns served to identify the troops to each other following the US-led coalition's invasion of Iraq in 2003.

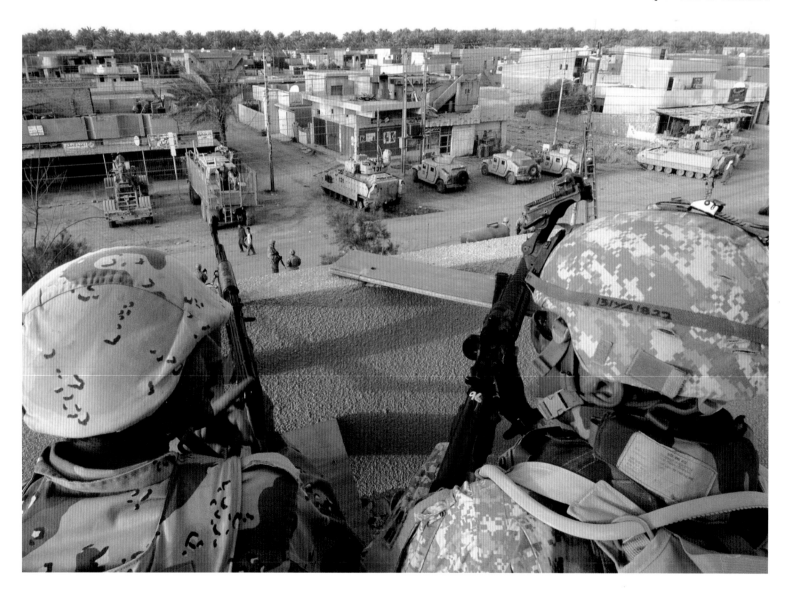

their national identity. In 1960, Poland introduced a leopard-skin pattern for its paratroopers – a deliberate historical reference to the panther skins worn by the elite 17th-century Polish Winged Hussars. Since the collapse of the Soviet Union in 1991, many neighbouring states to Russia have rushed to devise completely different military patterns to emphasize their distance from their former masters.

In the early 1970s, after a period of following its American allies, West Germany re-established itself as a camouflage pioneer by pursuing other nature-based patterns including a winter pine-needles motif. The *Flecktarnmuster* – four-colour clusters of small blobs – became the combat uniform of a reunited Germany in 1990, but its resemblance to wartime Waffen-SS patterns had alienated some NATO allies who had tested it in the 1980s. The Dutch army dropped it and replaced it with a pattern similar to British DPM.

That the choice of camouflage patterning could be a controversial political statement was demonstrated when some Arab nations adopted Nazi-style 'oak-leaf' and 'plane-tree' patterns in their wars against Israel. From 1975 onwards, Egyptian soldiers were ordered to wear more neutral designs.

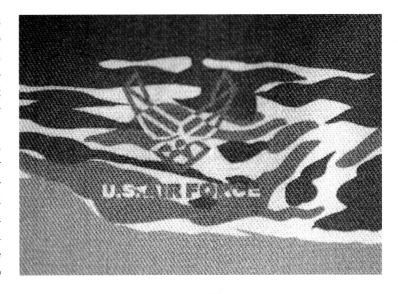

◤ **US Air Force insignia** incorporated into a new camouflage pattern, 2002.

◣ **US Marine Corps label** on new MARPAT ('Marine Pattern') camouflage combat dress, 2006.

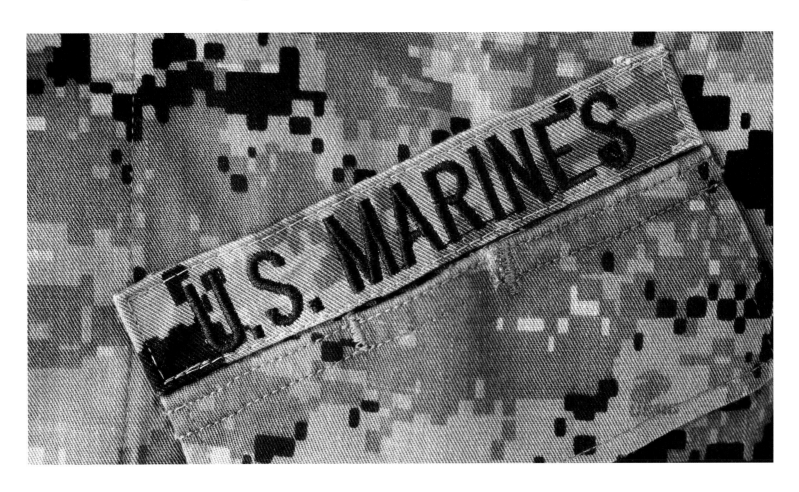

▲ **M62 Jacket, Finland**. This style of camouflage was adopted by the Finnish army from 1962 and used until 1991.

◤ **Soviet Russian summer field dress jacket.** This pattern, known as KLMK, was initially used by snipers, but was then issued to Soviet ground forces from the mid-1980s.

▷ **Australian army jacket, 1989 pattern**. Often known as 'jellybean' or 'ozcam', this pattern is made up of five colours designed to be suitable for all operations throughout the seasons in arid, desert, temperate and jungle regions.

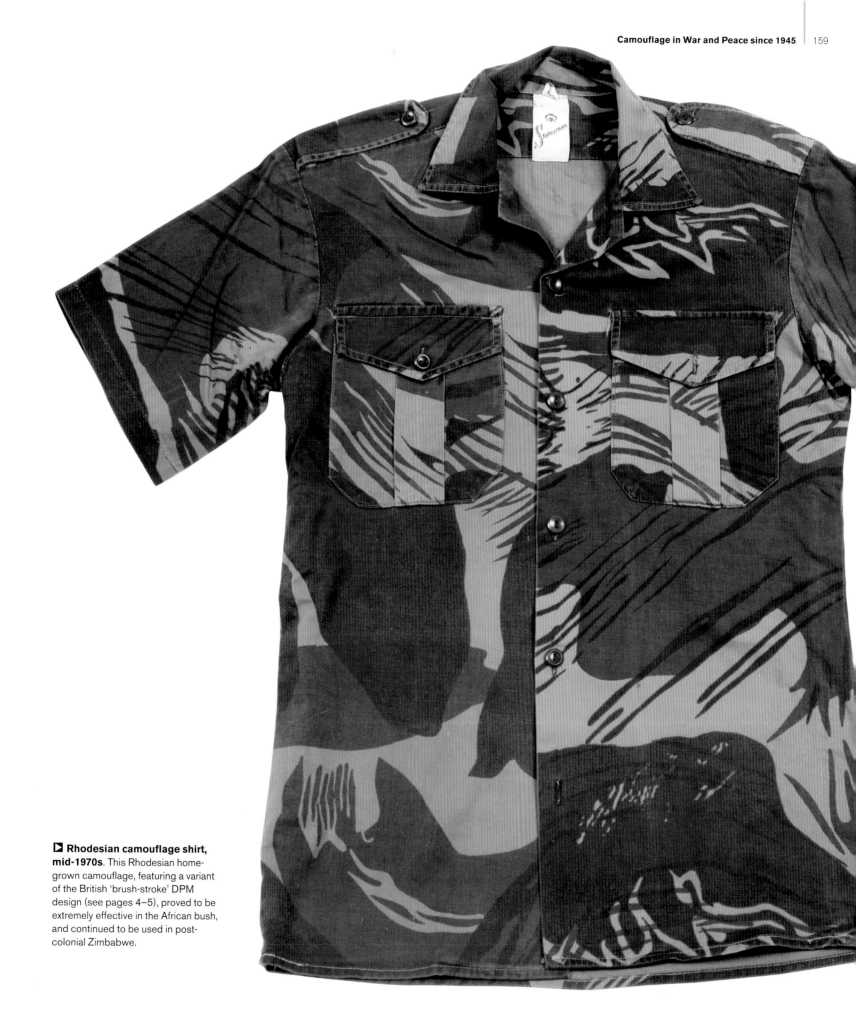

▶ **Rhodesian camouflage shirt, mid-1970s**. This Rhodesian home-grown camouflage, featuring a variant of the British 'brush-stroke' DPM design (see pages 4–5), proved to be extremely effective in the African bush, and continued to be used in post-colonial Zimbabwe.

The Future of Camouflage

Ever since the Second World War, camouflage manufacturers have been forced to consider the non-visual battlefield as well as the visual landscape. Infrared reflectant dyes were incorporated in German and US camouflage suits as early as the 1940s.

By the 1980s, 'Stealth' technologies had made possible dramatic reductions in the visibility of military aircraft and vehicles to radar and other detection methods. Using a combination of sophisticated radar-absorbing materials and faceted surfaces, Stealth can reduce the radar signature of an aircraft to almost nothing. Its most famous deployment was on the US F-117A fighter-bomber. Colonel Barry Horne of the US Air Force knew it was working when he walked into a hangar on a Saudi Arabian air base during the Gulf War of 1991. 'In the mornings we'd find bat corpses littered around our air-planes inside the open hangars,' he recalled. 'Bats use a form of sonar to "see" at night, and they were crashing blindly into our low-radar-cross-section tails.'

Thermal Imaging technology, which detects body heat, is now the biggest threat to the individual soldier seeking to remain concealed. Camouflage scientists are attempting to reduce this heat signature in two main ways, either by deceiving the detector or by reducing the overall body heat of a soldier.

Shiny, metallic surfaces emit heat more slowly, so that if a layer of shiny material is sandwiched between traditional camouflage cloth, a Thermal Imager will only see the shiny surface and be deceived into detecting a lower heat signature.

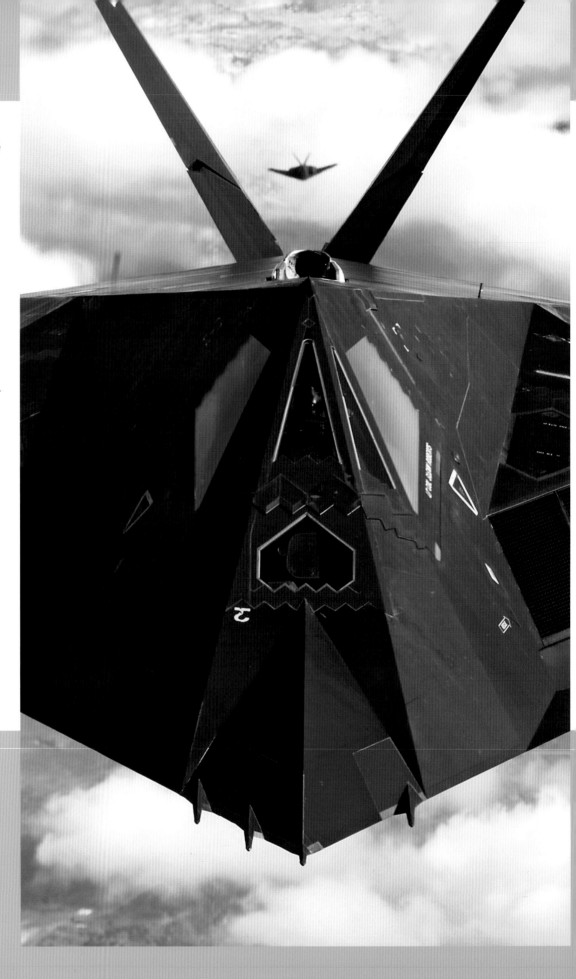

▶ **US F-117A Nighthawk Stealth fighter plane.** Developed during the Cold War as a weapon able to defy enemy radar, it spearheaded airstrikes against Iraq during the 1991 Gulf War with its laser-guided bombs.

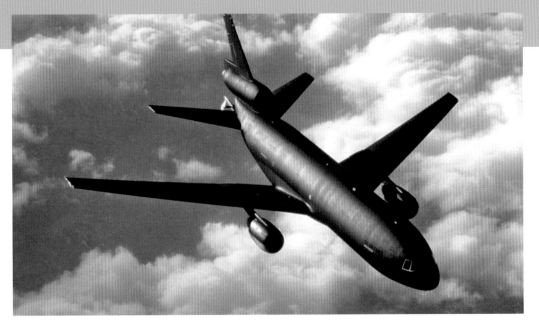

▲ **KC-10 tanker aircraft** which refuels the B-2 bomber in-flight, enabling it to reach around the globe.

▽ **The American B-2 Spirit** is protected from enemy detection by its use of Stealth design and materials.

A shiny, transparent visor could also shield a soldier's face. However, reducing heat loss in such ways could make the soldier uncomfortable, unless he was also fitted with a temperature-control system integrated into his combat suit.

Another method for defeating Thermal Imaging is one inspired by nature. The greater a body's surface area, the quicker it releases heat – the best example being an elephant's huge ears. By cladding a soldier in a uniform with fins or hanging strips of material, his body heat would be dissipated more efficiently and his temperature closer to that of his environment. But such a solution would have a revolutionary impact on the appearance of soldiers, not to mention being impractical to wear, and so probably would be unacceptable to them.

A variant on Stealth technology has been discovered by Spectro Dynamic Systems of North Carolina. Using a by-product of coal ash, they have produced a paint that contains microscopic ceramic balls coated with silver. This has proved a brilliant shield against electro-magnetic interference. The paint can be applied to a tank or mixed into fabric to make a combat jacket. Used in treated clothes or as face paint, it makes the wearer invisible to Thermal Imaging. A canvas cover treated with the paint has been used by US Special Forces to cloak the hot engines of their high-speed raiding boats.

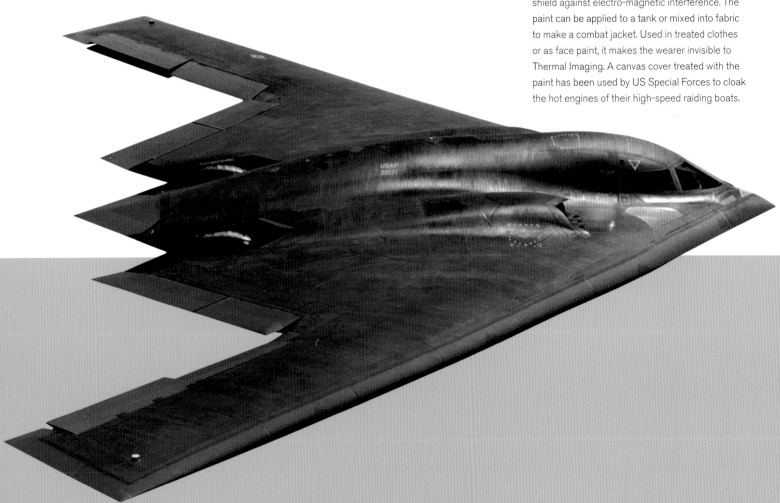

Scientists looking for more effective forms of military camouflage clothing have followed with interest new developments in high-tech textiles. In research funded by Mitsubishi Rayon in Japan, textile designer Sarah Taylor devised a tartan fabric using fibre optics that emanate light. Taylor wove the fibres into a cloth that sparkles when connected to a light source. The Defence Clothing and Textiles Agency in Colchester immediately saw its potential. If the fibre optics could be used to light up a fabric, they could also be used to produce more subtle forms of environmental colouring that could change to suit any landscape – a real chameleon textile.

Another line of research in 1998 was inspired by butterfly wings. Scientists have been studying the wing structure of certain species of butterfly to see how similar forms could be used to make soldiers and their vehicles almost invisible. Thousands of tiny scales on their wings create vivid, iridescent colours by bouncing light waves off their different surfaces, an effect known as interference. Scientists believe they could create butterfly suits for soldiers made from a multi-layered fibre that could be electronically adjusted to change colour.

In 2006, Sir John Pendry, professor of theoretical physics at Imperial College London, announced the possibility of creating an 'invisibility' cloak for military objects. Most materials are either opaque or transparent, either absorbing light photons or letting them pass through. But, in research funded partly by the Pentagon, Pendry and his colleagues discovered a third kind of material that can 'grab' photons without absorbing or allowing them through. These metallic materials carry the photons within themselves, then emit them the other side, as though they have passed through something transparent. Such a material could be used to coat warships or tanks to make them seem invisible.

'We know cloaking can be done with radar waves,' said Pendry. 'Light waves are another form of electromagnetic radiation, so making a material capable of cloaking against light should be possible within a decade.'

With such a camouflage, soldiers and their weapons would become truly invisible.

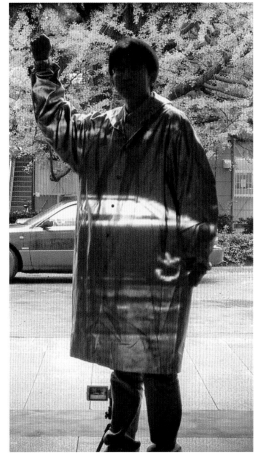

◿ **Real-life 'invisibility cloak'** designed by Masahiko Inami, Naoki Kawakami, and Susumu Tachi at the University of Tokyo in 2003. A man wears a reflective cape onto which is projected footage taken from a video camera of the scene behind him, creating the illusion of transparency.

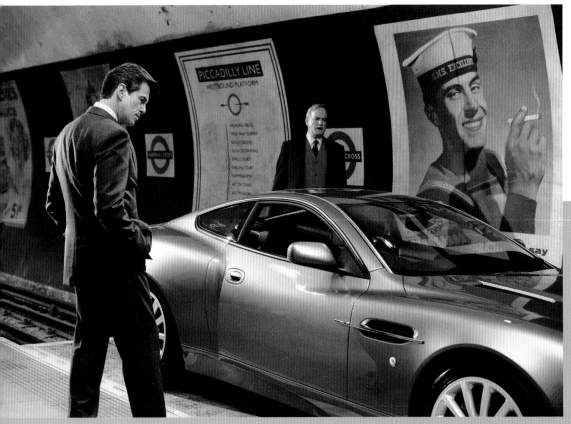

◿ **'Invisible' Aston Martin** from the James Bond film *Die Another Day*, 2002. In the film, the car has cameras and video screens attached to the bodywork which relay real-time images from one side of the vehicle to the other. The effect is to make it appear invisible from a variety of angles. Such technology is no longer entirely fictional; it has been tested in actual experiments.

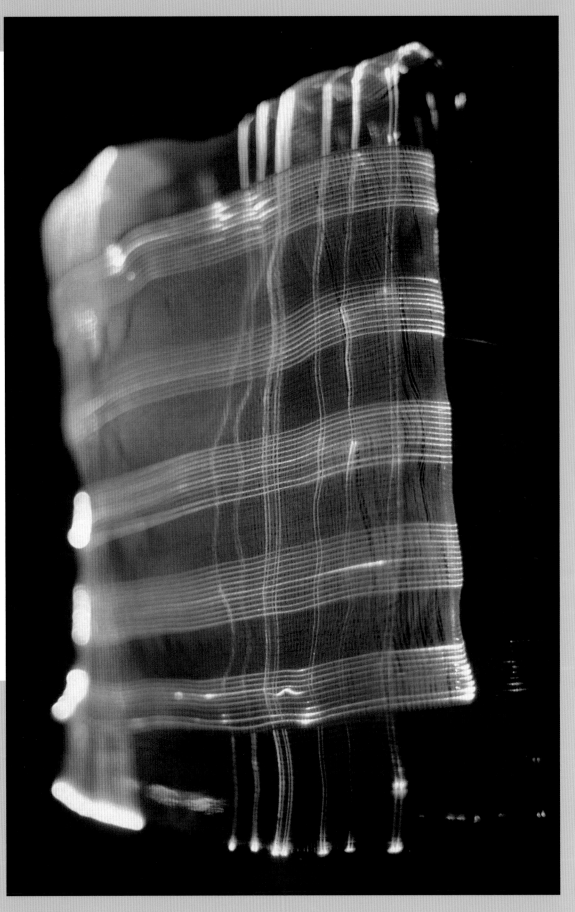

▶ **British designer Sarah Taylor** developed a tartan fabric woven with fibre optics that sparkle when connected to a light source. The next step for such technology may be a fabric that can change colours to reflect its environment.

▼ **Camoglaze, one-way visibility camouflage for car windscreens,** devised by Australian company Camtech. Similar to window tinting, Camoglaze also cuts glints from vehicle windows and comes in a removable version for windscreens.

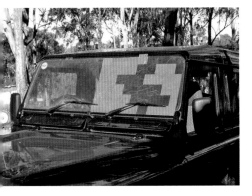

Camouflage in Protest, Art and Fashion

With the wide adoption of camouflage clothing by US and British soldiers, camouflage patterning entered the popular imagination. In the political turbulence of the later 1960s, it also came to be associated with protest and anti-establishment movements. One reason for this was that it was often worn by anti-war protesters and groups such as Vietnam Veterans Against the War. For many sympathetic artists and designers it was also a new symbol of militarism crying out to be subverted in anti-military protest art. At the height of student demonstrations in Paris in 1968, artist Pierre Buraglio produced *Mondrian Camouflaged*, a copy of one of Piet Mondrian's famous abstract grid compositions that inserted camouflage patterns in place of the coloured squares.

Other artists saw camouflage in a wider context of nature and history. Vera Lehndorff was a successful fashion model in the 1960s

▷▷ **The wearing of camouflage** clothing by anti-war protesters in the early 1970s helped camouflage enter the popular imagination and become part of the 'radical chic' of the period.

▽ **Camouflage-clad leaders** of Vietnam Veterans Against the War, who seized and occupied the Statue of Liberty for three days in December 1971 in opposition to the Vietnam War.

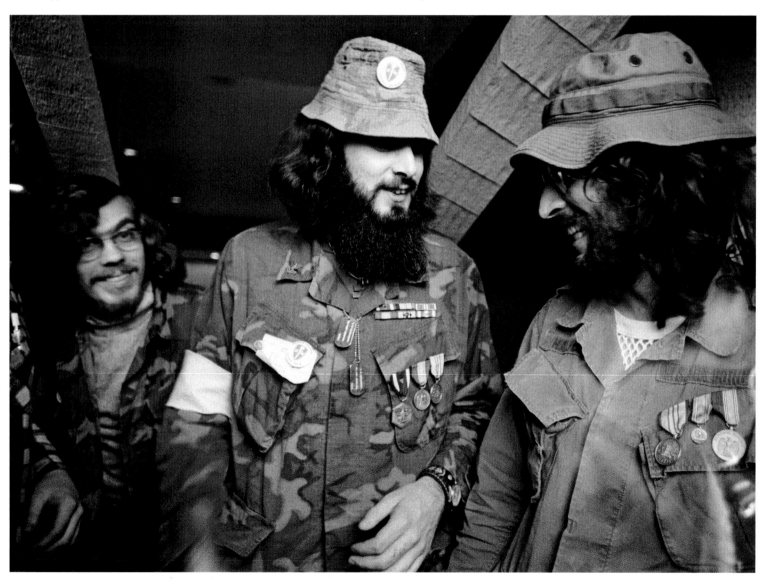

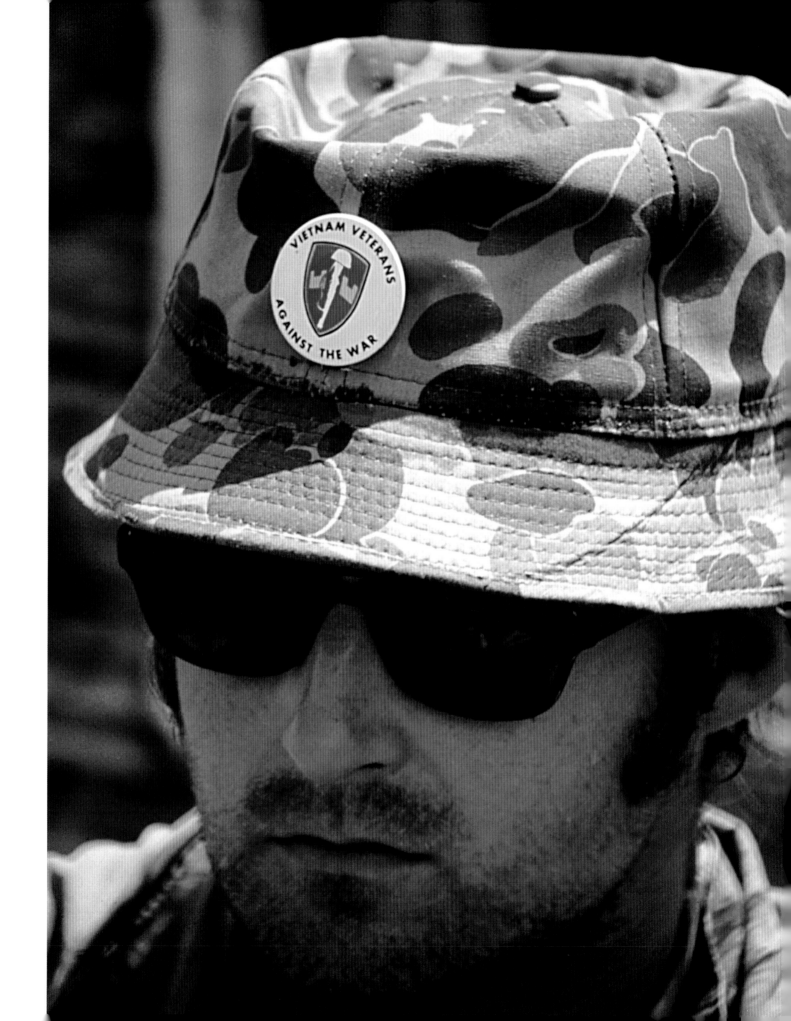

▶▶ **Camouflage suit made by** New York fashion designer Stephen Sprouse in 1987 using a pattern created by Andy Warhol, who experimented with camouflage to produce a series of paintings and prints the year before his death in 1987.

▶ *Iron Beam with Socket and Light Switch*, part of the *Oxidisation* series of 1978, a collaboration between photographer Holger Trülzsch and artist Vera Lehndorff (also known as the fashion model Veruschka). Lehndorff's naked body was painted to merge into a variety of backdrops, including the rusting pipework of this industrial building, in an exploration of the themes of camouflage and disguise.

▼ *Stone head*, Veruschka's earliest camouflage concept, 1969. Photograph by Rubartelli.

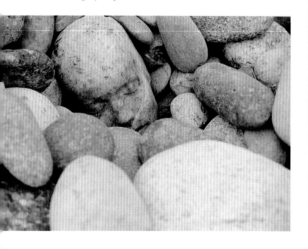

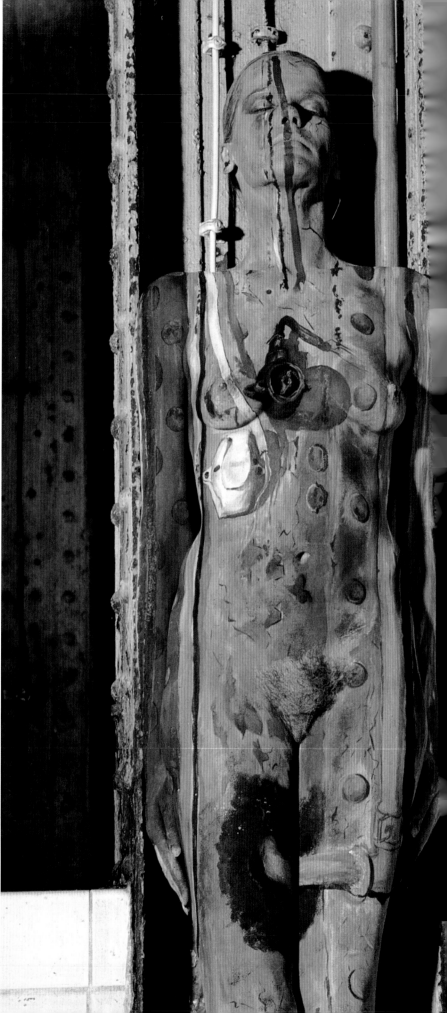

– working under the name Veruschka – but she had studied art as a student and returned to painting at the end of the decade. Her chosen canvas was her own body and she embarked on a quest to explore all different types of camouflage. It began one day while sitting on a terrace admiring some large stones. She painted her own head to look like a stone and then was photographed with just her head showing among a collection of the pebbles. It was a stark image of detachment that gave expression to some of the reasoning behind her art.

'As a model I could transform myself into many different characters,' she later wrote. 'Soon I began to paint myself as different animals and plants, knowing that they are often more beautiful then we are. The nakedness of human skin always disturbed me. By painting myself I could create the illusion of having feathers, fur, scales or leaves…. Camouflaging myself also made me feel that the public could not trap me so easily.'

From 1969 through the 1970s, Lehndorff worked with German photographer Holger Trülzsch to produce a series of remarkable images on the theme of camouflage painted on her naked body. At first, they copied boldly disruptive schemes from animals such as birds or antelope. Then they explored imagery incorporating man-made elements such as Renaissance grotto statuary overgrown with grass and moss. Finally, they embarked on a project altogether more surreal, painting her body to resemble parts of buildings so that her skin merged with the crumbling plaster of a cottage wall and a weathered window, or a rusting factory door complete with bolts and iron pipes.

The simple beauty of camouflage patterning, rather than its political symbolism, appealed immensely to the artist Andy Warhol. In 1986, a year before his death, he produced a series of prints and paintings based on the four-colour US M81 Woodland camouflage, which had become the standard pattern for US Army battle dress in the early 1980s. He painted it in traditional greens, browns and blacks, but also created versions in garish pinks, yellows and blues. He also produced a self-portrait with camouflage obscuring his face. In 1987 fashion designer Stephen Sprouse took some of Warhol's camouflage patterns and reproduced them on clothes – a very early example of the use of camouflage in high fashion.

In the meantime, camouflage patterns were being seized upon and reinvented in the world of street fashion. By the mid-1980s, two key US pop sub-cultures had adopted camouflage. Hip hop bands were wearing military-style clothing, including camouflage, as part of their urban warfare look. New York-based hip hop artists Public Enemy wore a black and white urban version of the Woodland pattern to promote their seminal 1988 album *It Takes a Nation of Millions to Hold Us Back*. At the same time, in

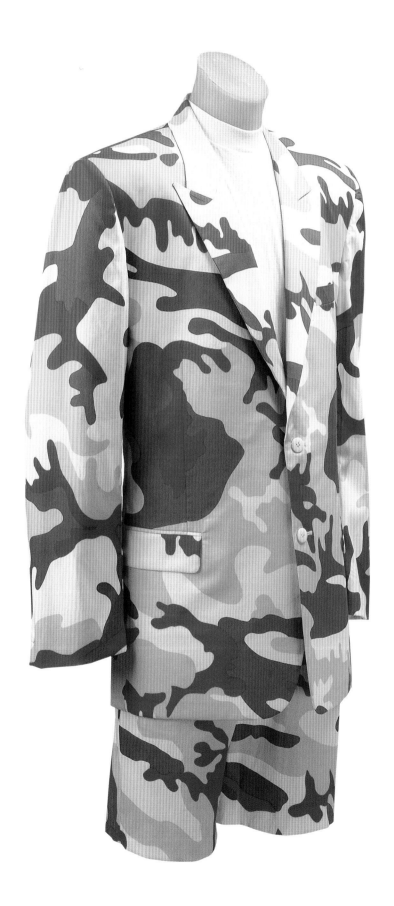

gay pop culture originating in San Francisco and New York, military clothing had long been one of a range of 'macho' looks worn in the clubs.

Both these sub-cultures provided sounds that went mainstream in the late 1980s and became part of a wave of enormously popular dance music that dominated the next decade. Their styles were adopted alongside their music throughout the Western world. By the mid-1990s, camouflage clothes, and especially camouflage combat trousers, were highly popular street fashion around the world. The most popular patterns were US Woodland, US Desert chocolate-chip, British DPM, and a Swiss red *Leibermuster*-style pattern.

The appeal of 'camo' was rooted in its counter-culture associations. This was clothing that was definitely not inspired by high fashion, but was coming from the streets. It was anti-fashion in the

▶▶ **Members of hip hop** band Public Enemy in black and white urban versions of US Woodland pattern camouflage, 1987.
Photography © GLEN E. FRIEDMAN.
Reprinted with permission from the Burning Flags Press book *FUCK YOU HEROES* (www.BurningFlags.com)

▼ **British pop band the Eurythmics** in concert at Bercy, Paris, in 1999. Annie Lennox and Dave Stewart wear suits by Richard James made of British DPM camouflage.

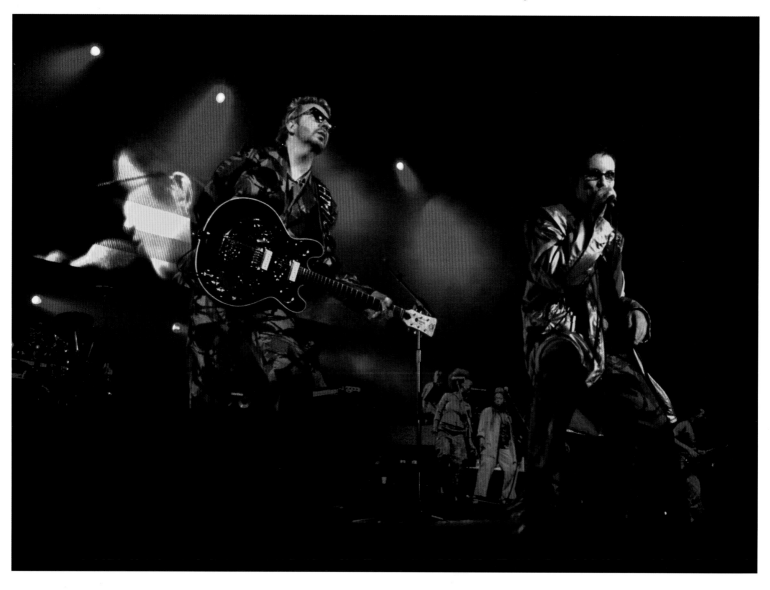

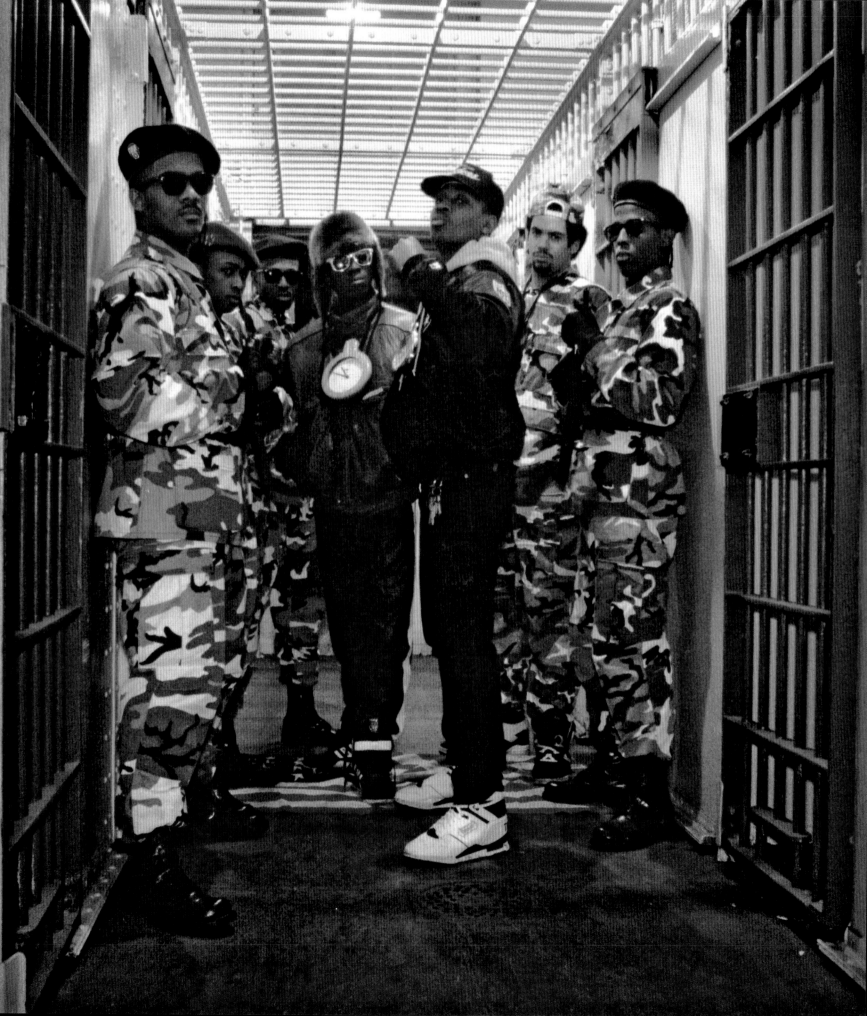

way that denim jeans once were before they became universally acceptable. The appeal of military-style clothing was that it was both aggressive and utilitarian.

Always ready to borrow from street fashion, high fashion designers were also excited by camouflage and by the mid-1990s had jumped on the popular trend, adapting patterns to all kinds of couture clothing and accessories. British designer Paul Smith invented his own version of camouflage by using photographic prints of green ivy on zip-up jackets and accessories. Italian fashion house Versace created a camouflage suit. French fashion house Louis Vuitton put the chic Swedish pink-coin pattern on raincoats. High fashion interest in camouflage has proceeded in cycles but it is still present over a decade after its first impact.

British fashion designer Hardy Blechman has explored camouflage more thoroughly than any other contemporary designer. Blechman began his Maharishi label in 1996 by recycling and reinventing army surplus clothing (see page 149), becoming fascinated by its utilitarian design and the quality of the materials. In his own designs he first used camouflage trim and then moved on to creating camouflage patterns of his own. These deliberately subvert the military associations of camouflage, incorporating symbols of nature and peace – for example the ancient *om* motif, ganja leaves and smoke trails, temples, dragons and bonsai trees growing from heavenly clouds.

'In the 1990s,' says Blechman, 'our perception of camouflage finally changed. It was no longer about concealment, but became a symbol. Civilians are attracted to it not because of its military context, but because it represents something else. With its organic shapes and natural colouring, it represents landscape and nature. It has become for many, unconsciously, a first step towards spiritual renewal.'

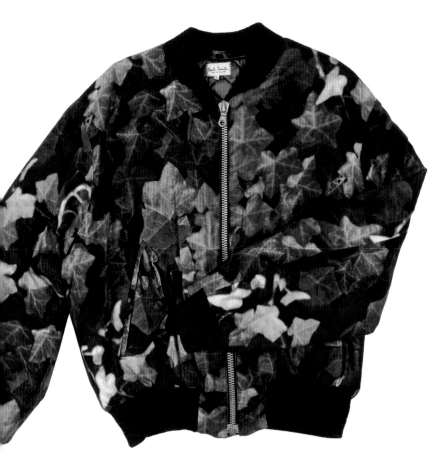

◨ ◧ **Jacket and handbag designed** by Paul Smith with his own camouflage pattern of ivy leaves. From the Paul Smith autumn/winter 2003 collection.

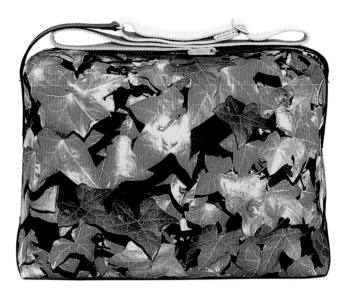

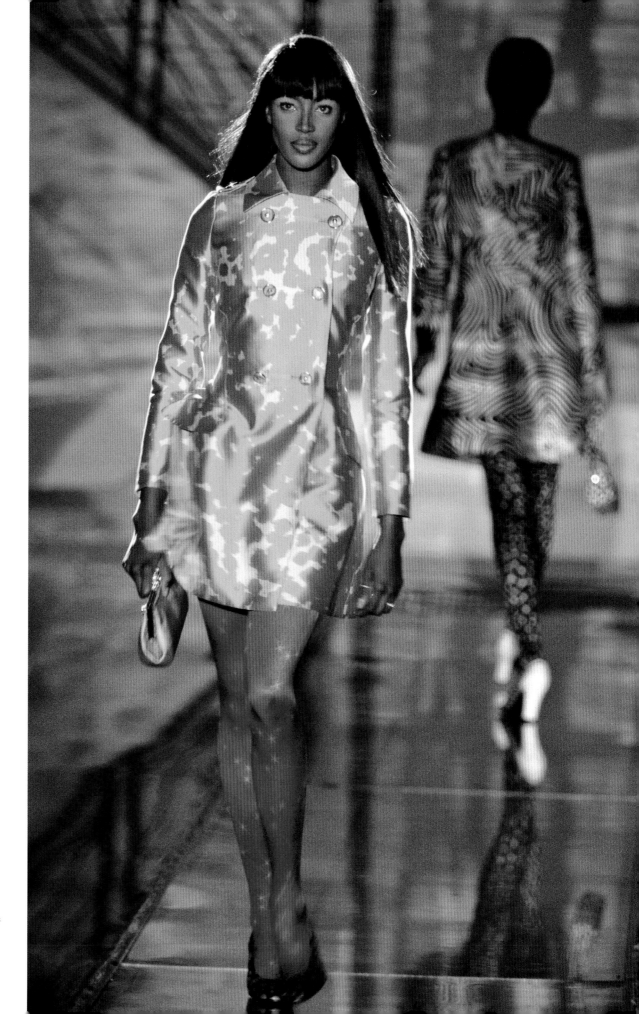

▶ **In the 1990s, high fashion** picked up the trend for wearing camouflage prints and applied them to some startling designs, such as this Versace dress modelled by Naomi Campbell in 1996.

▶ **Japanese designer Yohji Yamamoto** created this camouflage dress for his spring 2006 collection.

▼ **Camouflage dress by Italian designer Valentino Garavani**, part of his 1994 autumn/winter haute couture collection, modelled by Claudia Schiffer.

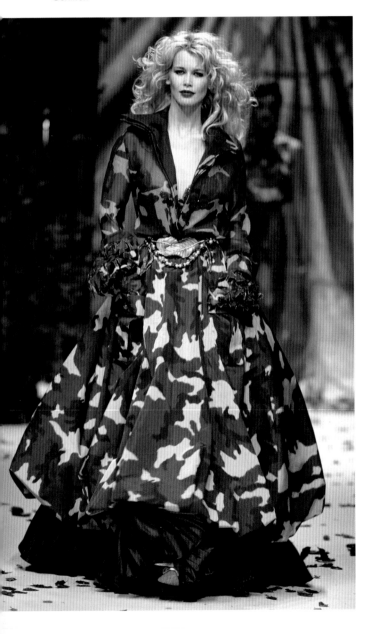

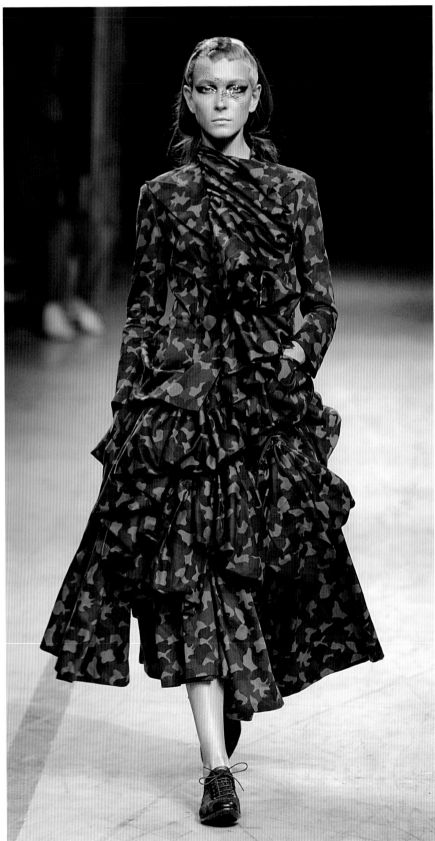

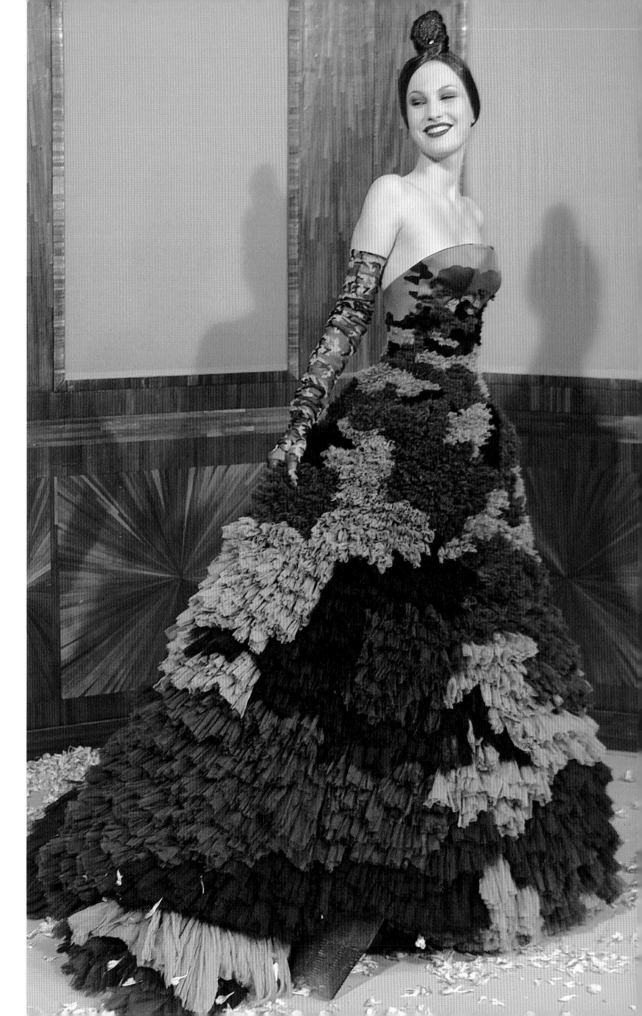

▶ **French designer Jean Paul Gaultier** caused a stir with this extravagant camouflage chiffon gown, part of his spring/summer 2000 collection.

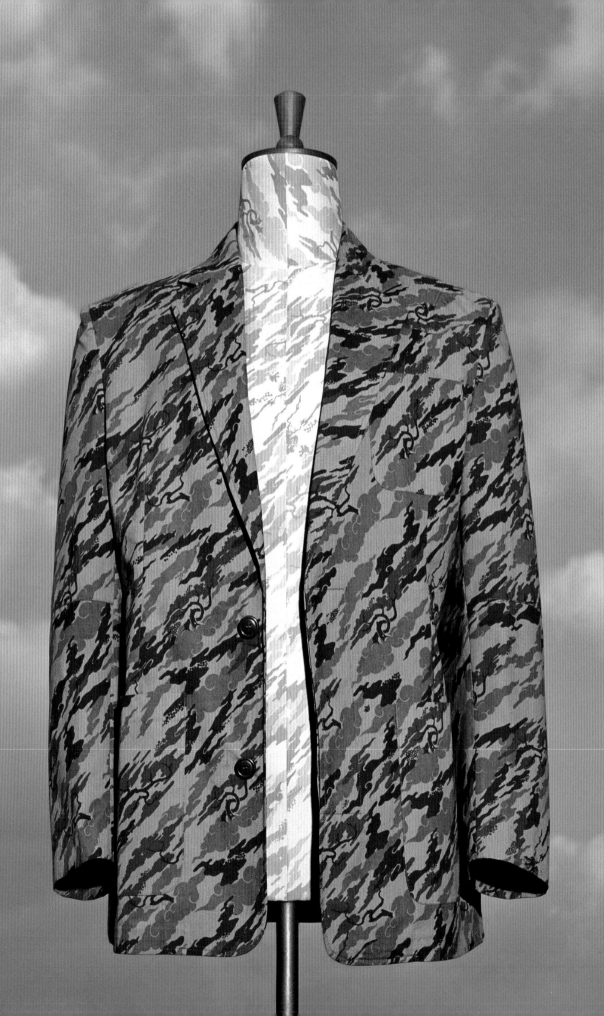

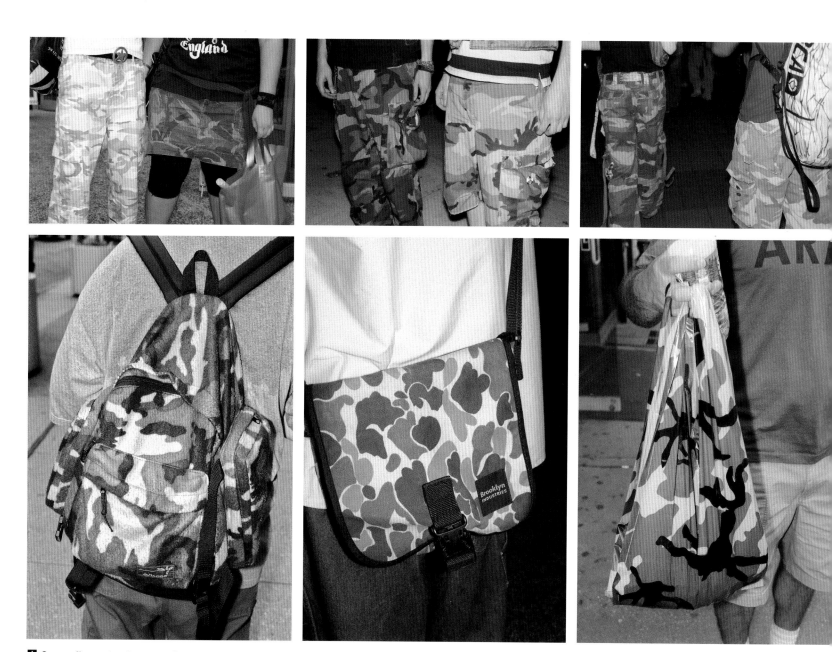

△ **Camouflage streetwear and accessories** photographed by Theodore Coulombe. By the 1990s, camouflage had become a global trend.

◁ **British designer Hardy Blechman** has become one of the most innovative adapters of camouflage to civilian fashion through his Maharishi label. His own camouflage patterns, such as 'Bonsai Forest' which adorns this blazer from his spring/summer 2004 collection, reclaim camouflage from its military origins by bringing to it more peaceful images and associations.

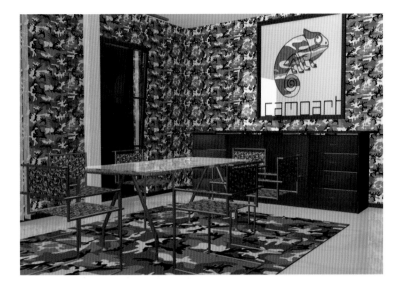

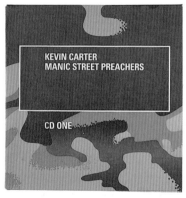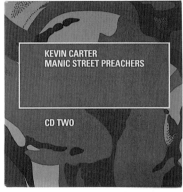

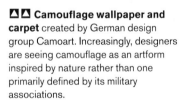 **Camouflage wallpaper and carpet** created by German design group Camoart. Increasingly, designers are seeing camouflage as an artform inspired by nature rather than one primarily defined by its military associations.

CD covers for a single released by Welsh rock band the Manic Street Preachers in 1996 about the death of war photojournalist Kevin Carter. They feature classic camouflage patterns redrawn by designer Mark Farrow.

The Universal Language of Camouflage

In the 1990s, camouflage became a fashionable decorative pattern beyond clothing, appearing on objects from mugs to pens to CD covers. Its aesthetic qualities began to be taken seriously by designers. Quentin Newark of London design group Atelier Works wrote an article on the subject in *Creative Review* in March 1997. He claimed camouflage was a major thread of organic design in an otherwise modernist, machine-led century and should form the basis of a new school of design that would move closer to nature. 'It is time for the rest of us to express our growing affinity and concern for nature,' he wrote. 'What better way to do this than in the way we dress and the forms we surround ourselves with?'

The association between camouflage and natural environments has helped to soften its martial image and made it far more acceptable in civilian life. Designers have used camouflage fabric as a covering for sofas, beds and soft furniture, and applied camouflage paint to tables, chairs and cabinets.

At the same time, the military context of camouflage continues to be a useful design short-hand. The rock group Manic Street Preachers employed camouflage patterns on their 1996 CD covers, redrawn by designer Mark Farrow, to invoke a military context for their single 'Kevin Carter', about the death of the young war photojournalist. Janice Kirkpatrick of Glasgow-based design group Graven Images created a series of posters about devolution in the United Kingdom in which she showed a disintegrating map of the regions of Scotland in camouflage colours. It inferred the threat of a civil war like that in the Balkans if nationalist politics were allowed to get out of hand.

By January 2001, the London *Evening Standard* reported that the global fashion for camouflage design was worth £1.5 billion a year. It quoted the US online store Out in Style as having sales of camouflage fashion accessories of £375,000, compared to £50,000 only three years previously. 'The word from the couture houses across the world is: Camo is hot and getting hotter all the time,' said the newspaper. 'In Germany the craze is for camouflage bedsheets. In France they go wild for camouflaged loo paper while in Belgium camouflage curtains are all *la rage*.' Even investment analysts on the Frankfurt stock exchange were commenting on its future potential for generating money.

But not everyone was impressed with camouflage fashion. A ten-year-old boy wearing camouflage T-shirt and trousers was stopped from entering Barbados on holiday with his parents in 1999. Airport police told him to take off his camouflage clothes or be sent back home. They explained it was against the law for anyone to wear camouflage clothing on the island, except for the Barbados Defence Force.

▼ Skateboards made by US company Powell-Peralta, a cult skateboarding brand. Their pattern indicates the continuing credibility and appeal of camouflage to youth sub-cultures.

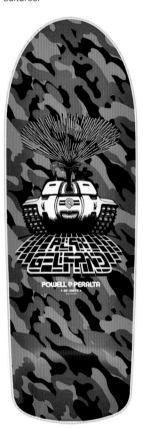

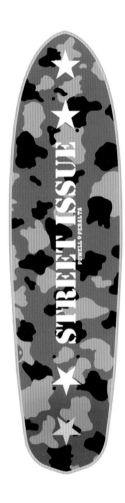

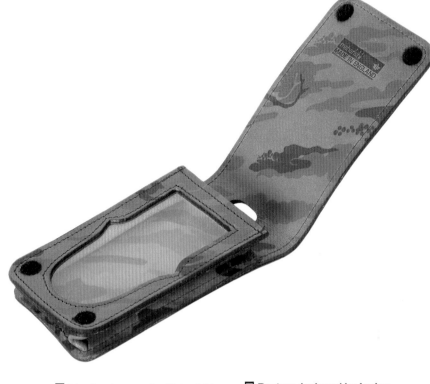

▲ I-Lectronics case by Maharishi featuring the label's Bonsai Forest pattern.

▼ Posters designed by Janice Kirkpatrick of Glasgow-based design group Graven Images. Part of a series, they express her reservations with the campaign for political devolution in the United Kingdom.

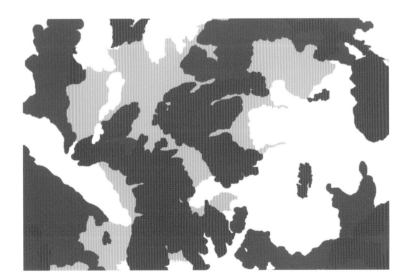

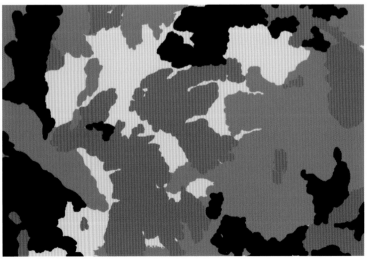

▶ *The Dark Side of Dazzle*,
installation in clay and wood, by Marilyn
Lysohir, 1985–86. A warship clad in
brilliant patterning expresses the artist's
ambivalence about such an application
of art. When exhibited at the Museum
of Art at Washington State University,
the installation was accompanied by
tape recordings of war stories.

Contemporary Artists Inspired by Camouflage

Almost a century after its first appearance in the
First World War, military camouflage continues to
excite artists all around the world. In much of this
work, it is the fact that camouflage has become a
signifier – rather than a deceiver – that most
interests the artist.

In 2003, as Western nations went to war in Iraq,
Arlene Elizabeth created an American flag out of
a myriad of origami cranes folded in camouflage-
patterned paper. 'The flag is represented as an
image floating in isolation against the sky,' she said,
'and all the cranes represent camouflage worn by
the US military. Usually, camouflage is employed
to hide or conceal a surface, but here it is used to
reveal a current underneath. Though it pained me
to make this, I do feel that this representation of the
flag is more in line with what the World sees when
we hoist the white-red-and-blue.' She called her
piece *Camouflage (The Color of Globalization)*.

Another American artist, Claire Lieberman,
prefers to use the language of Pop Art in her
references to camouflage. She has made bright,
fluorescent patterns out of Jello-O (see pages
146–47). The organic patterns clash with the
garish synthetic gleam of the man-made food. 'The
cheeriness of the colors,' said the catalogue of her
2005 Seattle exhibition, 'put one in mind of smiley
faces and Disneyland. Magic Kingdom indeed.'
US Woodland camouflage, it seems, is now as
identifiable with America as Mickey Mouse.

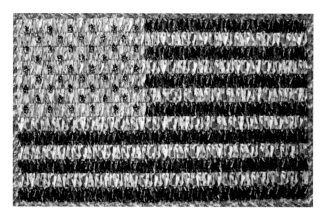

◀▼ *Camouflage: The Colour of
Globalization*, folded camouflage-
pattern paper, by Arlene Elizabeth,
2003 (left and detail below). Folded into
origami cranes, the sheets of paper are
printed with camouflage patterns worn
by US troops and arranged in the form
of an American flag.

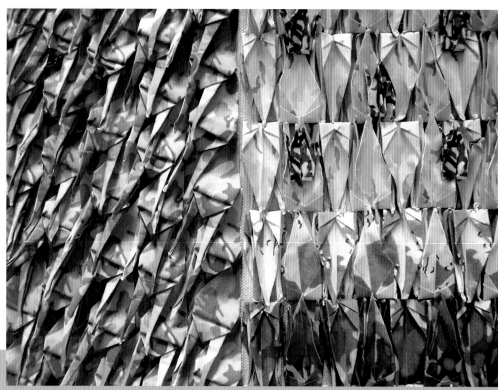

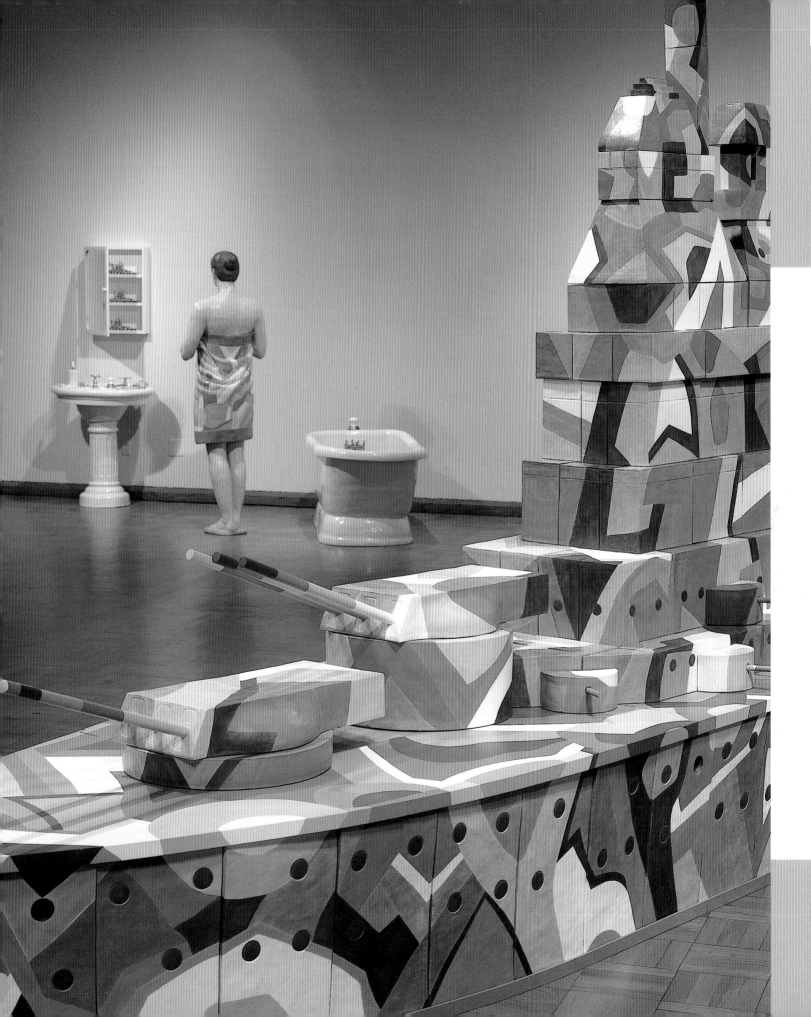

▼ ***True Colours***, photography and video by Juan Pedro Fabra Guemberena, 2002. These figures are so closely identified with their setting that they have the air of natural spirits emerging out of the landscape.

▼ ***pbf!pbf!pbf!pbf!***, enamel on aluminium by Ingrid Calame, 2002. Her apparently foliage-filled abstract landscapes are in fact generated from the shapes of random stains traced from pavements around her studio.

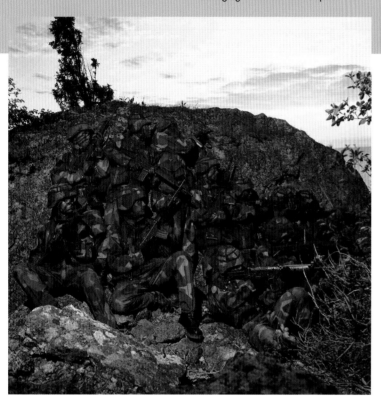

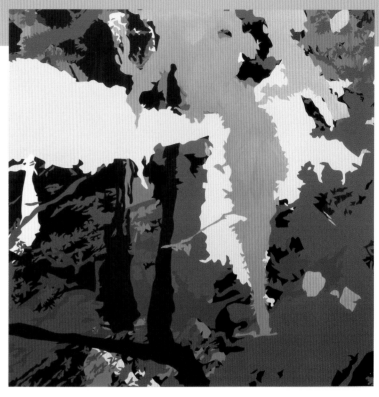

In photographs and videos, Uruguayan artist Juan Pedro Fabra Guemberena has explored the idea of camouflage as a symbol of nature. In *True Colours* (2002), he posed several models in full camouflage combat uniform against a Danish landscape so they looked as though they had grown out of it. 'The soldiers increasingly resemble some kind of phantom figures of the forest,' said critic Rodrigo Mallea Lira, 'like trolls or spirits.'

Los Angeles-based Ingrid Calame paints shiny enamel on aluminium to create sensuous landscapes that evoke both Henri Rousseau's jungle paintings and the abstract expressionism of Jackson Pollock. With titles such as *p-cheew-chtu-chtu* and *eee-rr…pffp*, these use the splodges and the foliage-like shapes of camouflage patterns to make magnificently complex and strange landscapes. Many of these random shapes derive from stains and marks traced from pavements near her studio. Calame reproduces each mark in a single colour, creating an enormously rich mesh of shapes that begin to form landscapes in the viewer's mind.

Other artists reject the symbolism of camouflage and enjoy the pure aesthetic pleasure of its organic forms. When cartoonist Gerald Scarfe was invited to design the sets and costumes for the English National Ballet's production of *The Nutcracker* in 2002, he chose camouflage as a dominant design element. Some dancers were dressed in black-and-white Dazzle patterns, including coloured hair, while the Nutcracker Prince wore a magnificent jacket of red and gold camouflage splodges against a white background.

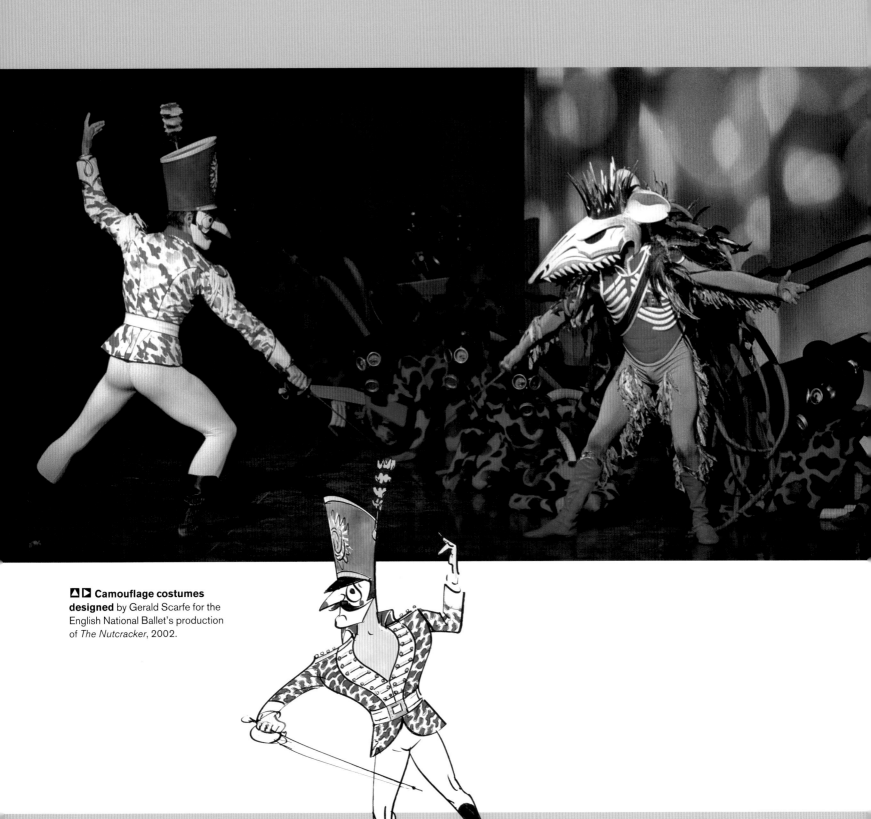

◤▶ Camouflage costumes designed by Gerald Scarfe for the English National Ballet's production of *The Nutcracker*, 2002.

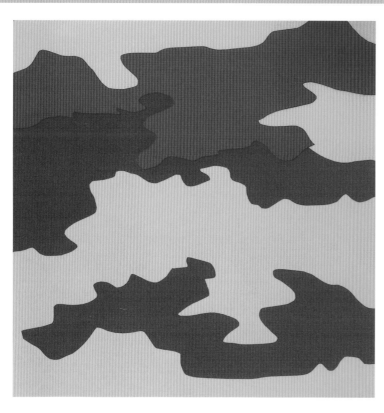

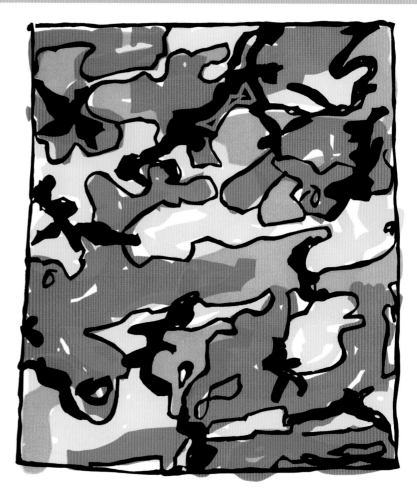

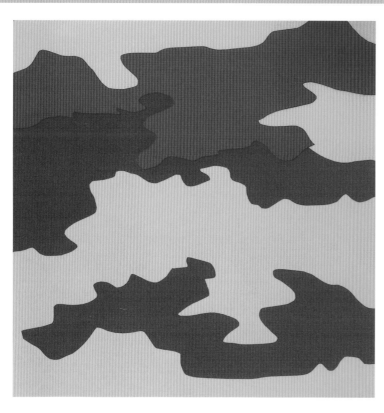 ◪ *Las Vegas (Red Rock Canyon)*, acrylic on canvas, by Tim Newark, 2002. Newark takes inspiration from specific landscapes and settings to create new versions of classic camouflage patterns. He believes 'every city, every neighbourhood should have its own camouflage pattern'.

▶ *Camouflage Jell'O II*, four-colour linoleum cut printed in fluorescent inks by Claire Lieberman, 2005. The Day-Glo colours of her patterns turn on its head the military idea of camouflage as concealment or disguise.

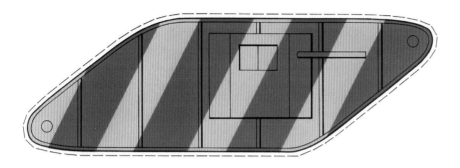

NECKTANK (1918)

IAN HAMILTON FINLAY/MICHAEL HARVEY · WILD HAWTHORN PRESS

◀ *NeckTank (1918)*, lithograph by Ian Hamilton Finlay with Michael Harvey, 1973. Exploring the tension between the decorative qualities of camouflage and the menacing nature of the military equipment to which it is applied, the artists have devised their own camouflage for a First World War British Mark IV tank.

◢ *Arcadia*, lithograph by Ian Hamilton Finlay with George Oliver, 1973. Here the artists have applied a leaf-pattern camouflage design to a Second World War German Panzer III tank.

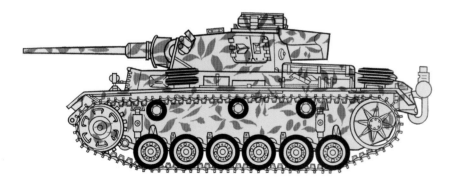

ARCADIA

IAN HAMILTON FINLAY/GEORGE OLIVER · WILD HAWTHORN PRESS

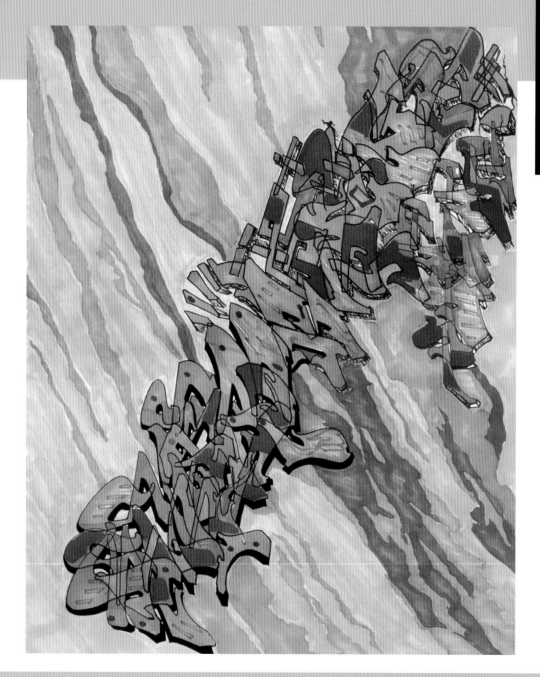

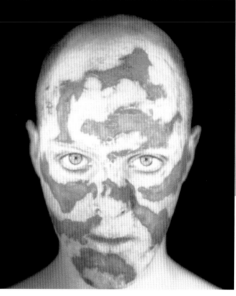

🔺 *Camouflage (Self-Portrait)*, photograph by Gavin Turk, 1998. Camouflage as birthmark or tattoo.

◀ *Stylers of the Storm*, marker pen on paper, by Aaron 'Sharp' Goodstone, 2004. Sharp began as a New York graffiti artist and has gone on to have his work exhibited in galleries around the world.

▶ *Pink Tank*, painted by Aleksandra Mir and others, photographed by Robin Sellick, 2002. This tank is a public artwork located in south London. Its colour echoes that of another famous tank originally mounted by the Soviets on a pedestal in Prague's central square after the crushing of the Prague Spring in 1968, supposedly as a memorial to the Russian soldiers who had liberated the population from the Nazis back in 1945, but in practice to remind the locals that Moscow didn't take kindly to anyone 'reforming' Communism. In 1991 it was painted pink by Czech artist David Cerny amid celebrations of the transformation from Soviet rule.

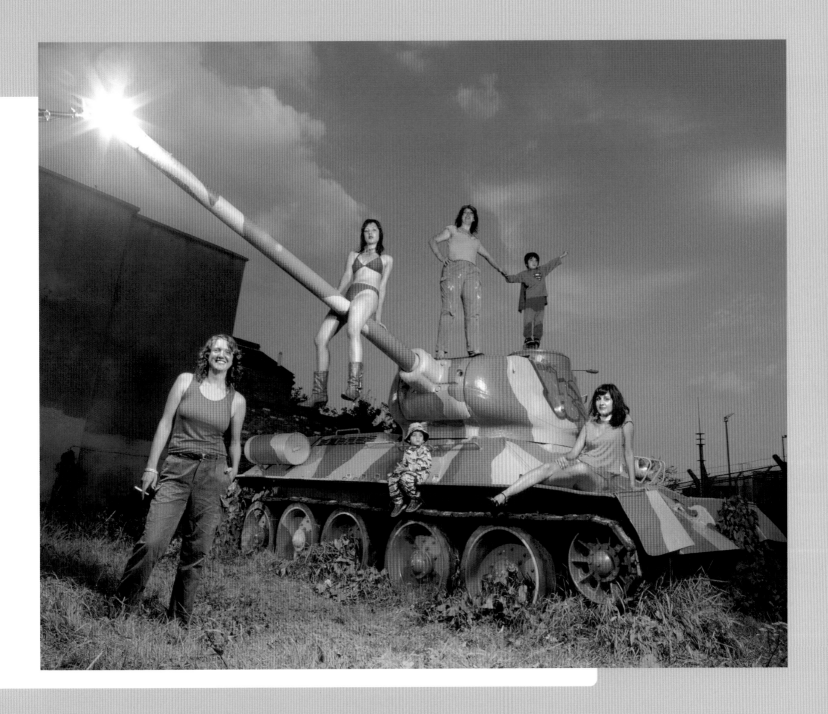

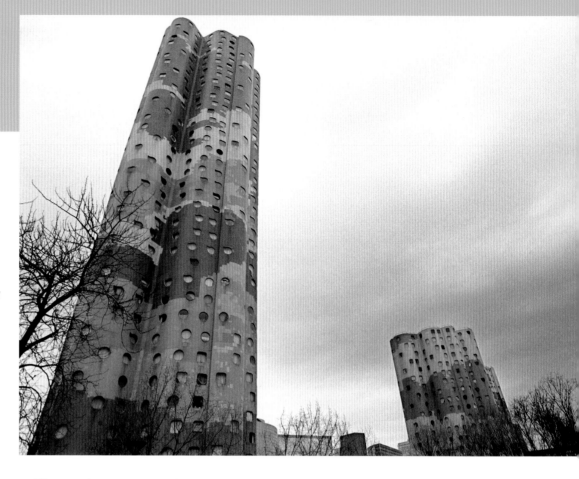

Camouflage Architecture

Prehistoric man lived in a variety of camouflaged dwellings, from tree-houses to cave shelters, to reed huts on stilts set among marshes. Made of local materials, they merged easily into the landscape and helped protect communities from other hunting groups. This tradition continues today among remote societies. With the development of more secure and complex societies in Europe and Asia, it became possible to create buildings from materials brought from far away, and architectural styles began to develop that spoke of bolder aspirations. In the West, the Classical and Gothic styles evolved, dominating European culture for over two thousand years. Here, the idea was not to hide, but to proclaim wealth, faith or power. But even in the Classical tradition, ideas of camouflaged architecture can be found.

In Renaissance gardens, designers sought to create an environment that referred to Greek and Roman myths and part of this fantasy was the grotto – a cave in which primeval forces could be appreciated. A grotto was a man-made structure, built to look like a real cavern, often with stalactites and stalagmites, or a stream running through it. It was intended to house dinner parties in which wealthy men and women could indulge more passionate interests beyond the civilized restraints of the classical palace. Outside, the rocky buildings were overgrown with plants and trees.

Twentieth-century Modernism, with its straight lines and clean facades, was no friend of organic design. The only time architecture met camouflage now was in war. But by the 1970s, environmental concerns led some architects to consider buildings that merged with the landscape rather than dominated it.

'We must make a peace treaty with nature,' declared Austrian artist Friedensreich Hundertwasser in 1983. 'We must restore to nature territories which we have illegally occupied.' To counter the brutality of Modernism, he imagined multi-storey buildings and public amenities such as car parks covered in layers of grass and trees. Following on from his ideas, a few private 'mole' houses were built as subterranean structures only open to the sky through ocular courtyards with the rest disguised underneath a mound of earth.

Environmental architecture was taken a step further by the Site group in the United States which conceived architectural projects in which buildings were smothered in plants. One watercolour sketch showed the New York skyline covered in foliage with vines streaming down from skyscrapers. Trained as artists rather than architects, the group's projects have mostly taken the form of visual studies only, but in 1992 they were commissioned to produce a building for the World Expo in Seville. The result was an undulating wall of glass with water flowing down it, encasing a restaurant and monorail station. They also used foliage and a vine-covered trellis to cover other buildings at the exhibition.

Postmodernist architecture, with its renewed interest in surface decoration, also found inspiration in camouflage. The intense, bright patterns used by Vienna-based practice Coop Himmelb(l)au on the Groninger Museum in the Netherlands have echoes of Dazzle, creating a blurring of form by visual over-stimulation. At La Défense in Paris, residential skyscrapers in 1977 were given a disruptive pattern of blue, grey, and brown by French architect Emile Aillaud, inspiring the nickname the *Tours Nuages* or 'Cloud Towers'.

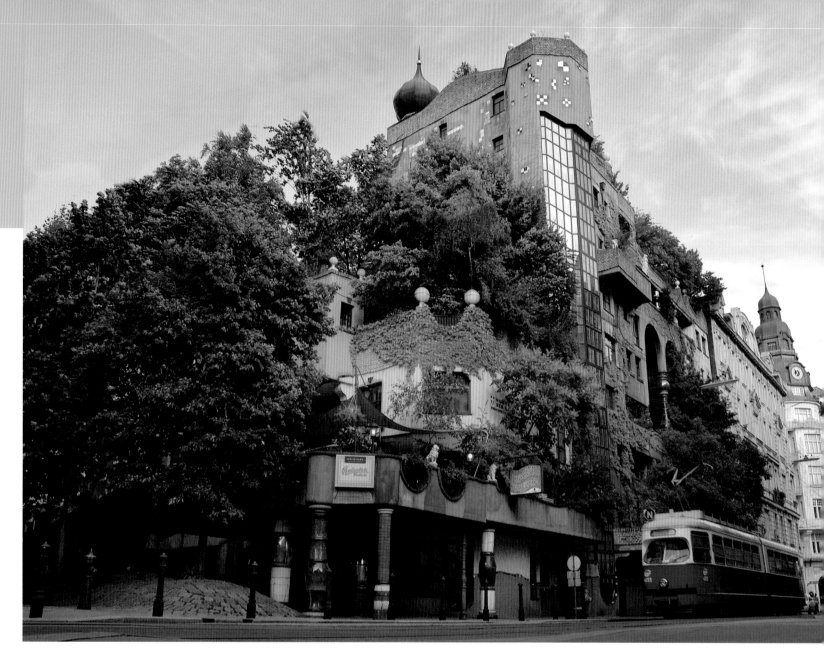

Residential skyscrapers at La Défense in Paris, erected in 1977. Their disruptive pattern decoration led to them being nicknamed the *Tours Nuages* or 'Cloud Towers'.

Hundertwasserhaus, **Vienna.** Austrian artist Friedensreich Hundertwasser was a pioneer in creating environmentally friendly architecture smothered in foliage. This extraordinary public-housing complex was erected in 1985.

The East Pavilion of the Groninger Museum in the Netherlands designed by Vienna-based architects Coop Himmelb(l)au, 1993–94. Constructed like the hull of a ship, the building's steel plates were decorated with a bold black and red disruptive pattern.

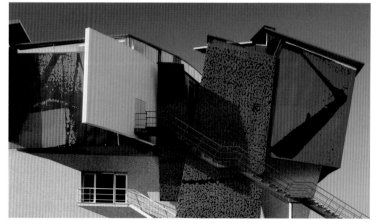

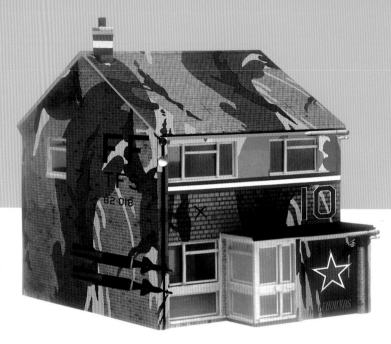

In 1998, the London design group FAT smothered a suburban house in khaki disruptive pattern plus painted missiles and weapons. At first, the result may appear to be an ironic statement on the use of camouflage as disguise given that such a decorated house would stand out absurdly on an estate of similar homes. But the intention was very serious.

'We were invited to contribute to an exhibition entitled *Utopia Revisited*,' said FAT group member Sam Jacob, 'the idea was to revitalize an estate of houses in east London by talking to the residents and asking them how they would like their houses to appear on the outside. Many of them suggested taking a hobby of the occupant and expressing that on the outside of the house, like golf or fishing. We took the idea of someone interested in military things.'

'You do not have to enter the language of contemporary architecture to make a significant building,' continued Jacob. 'You can use surface decoration — something that is underrated by serious modern architects — to make a difference and talk more in the language of ordinary people and their interests.'

With climate change becoming part of the political agenda in the West in the early 21st century, environmentally friendly architecture is referring back to much earlier lessons in camouflaged buildings. But it is not only the visible language of plant-covered roofs and turf walls that is being quoted; these new buildings must also perform in an invisible world by reducing carbon emissions. This is generating a revolution in environmentally friendly building materials that will reduce still further the impact of a building on the natural world — the perfect camouflage.

▲ ▼ **British suburban house** exterior and interior designed by London design group FAT in 1998. The intention was not to hide the house but to decorate it inside and out in a way that would express the interests of the resident.

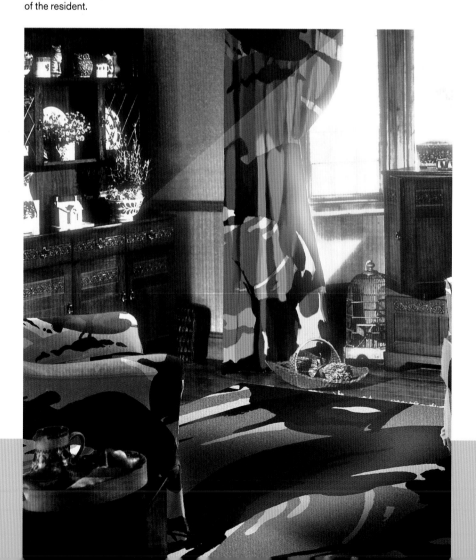

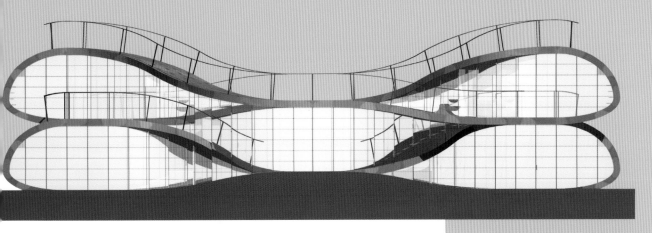

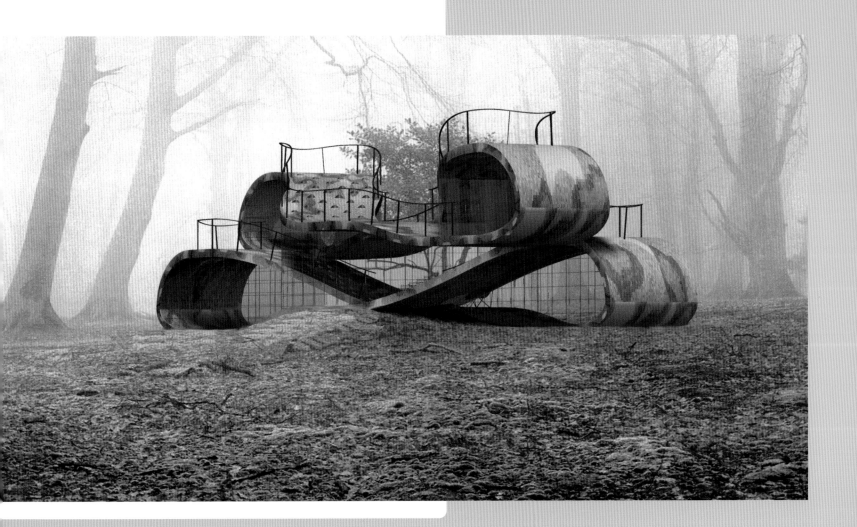

▲▼ *Virtual House* incorporating camouflage patterning designed by London-based Foreign Office Architects for a competition in 1997.

Acknowledgments

a = above, b = below, c = centre, l = left, r = right,

Imperial War Museum Collections 1 (UNI 12530), 8a (CT 792), 46a (UNI 2168), 52–53 (ART 2274), 54 (ART 5291), 55b (ART 5275), 58 (Q 8234, 82.72 Acc. No. K373000), 59 (K46964, ORD 108), 60 (ART 16369), 61 (ART 2283), 62 (ART 1152), 63 (Q 7878), 64 (Q 95957, Q95955), 68b (Q 17683), 69b (AIR 41), 70 (Q10058), 71 (ART 2965), 74b (IWM DAZ 0029 (1)), 75b (IWM DAZ 0029 (3)), 76–77 (MOD 2473, MOD 2471, MOD 2472, MOD 2474), 78 (ART 5728), 79 (ART 2293), 84 (UNI 010425, UNI 6062), 85 (Q 95964, Q 95965), 86 (EPHEM 307, EPHEM 306), 87 (Q 13392), 87b (UNI 8312), 90–91 (ART LD 141), 94l (EQU 1756), 95 (Major J Gray 83/38/ 1), 96r (83.9(41).0/5.5 Acc. No. 90/2334), 98 (both – Captain AE Havinden 74/165/8), 99 (Captain AE Havinden 74/165/8), 100 (H 3306), 101 (MOD 149), 102a (ART LD 1097), 103 (ART LD 2126), 104–105 (90 2334), 106–107 (Captain AE Havinden 74/165/8), 108 (ART LD 2757), 111 (ART LD 322), 112 (ART LD 3025, 113 (ART LD 3028, ART LD 3024), 114 (Major DAJ Pavitt 86/50/3), 115 (Captain AE Havinden 74/165/8), 116 (IWM Exhibits & Firearms Collection), 118 (83.9(41).0/5.5), 119 (E 008361, H 42527), 120–121 (ART LD 838), 121 (ART LD 1940), 122 (TR 1402, Sundour Collection), 123 (Captain AE Havinden 74/165/8), 124a (ART LD 1664), 124b (ART LD 3021), 125 (D 17196), 126b (90 2334 1 1), 127 (04(41):02.0/5 Acc. No. 84/615), 128–129 (ART LD 5378), 129 (ART 15284), 130 (UNI 3892), 131 (UNI 12188), 133 (EQU 2506), 134 (EQU 2532, UNI 5931), 135 (UNI 3546, UNI 3594, UNI 12311), 136 (UNI 3601), 137al (UNI 3599), 138 (Major DAJ Pavitt 86/50/3), 139 (VEH 85, 4100.95.1), 140 (VEH 68, 4501.50.1), 141 (MOD 393), 142b (ART LD 3979), 144–145 (2010.285.1, CH 8605, 2010.115.1, ART LD 2125, MOD 597), 150 (UNI 12151), 153r (UNI 5822), 154–155 (UNI 5818, UNI 12615, UNI 988, UNI 2626), 158–159 (UNI 5955, UNI 618, UNI 807, UNI 5334), 183 (IWM ART 15807, ART 15809).

akg-images 39, 41, 44, 48a, 49, 68a, 72; **Courtesy Musée de Bernay** 57; © **Yale Center for British Art, Paul Mellon Collection, USA/ Bridgeman Art Library, London** 42, 48b; **Courtesy Camoart, www.camoart.com** 176a; **Courtesy CamTech** 126a, 163l; **Carlton Television** 43b; **Dee Conway Ballet & Dance Picture Library** 181a; © **Michel Arnaud/CORBIS 171**; © **Photo B.D.V./CORBIS 172l**; © **Jeremy Bembaron/Sygma/CORBIS 168**; © **Tobias Bernhard/zefa/ CORBIS** 13; © **Bettmann/CORBIS** 151, 161a; © **W. Perry Conway/ CORBIS 25**; © **Raymond Gehman/CORBIS** 50b; © **Todd Gipstein/ CORBIS 2–3**; © **Naturfoto Honal/CORBIS** 32a; © **David Hosking/ Frank Lane Picture Agency/CORBIS** 14b; © **Dennis Johnson/ Papilio/CORBIS** 15; © **Steve Kaufman/CORBIS** 24r; © **JP Laffont/ Sygma/CORBIS** 164; © **George D. Lepp/CORBIS** 17; © **Renee Lynn/ CORBIS** 21; © **Wally McNamee/CORBIS** 165; © **Tim Page/CORBIS** 152; © **Matthieu Paley/CORBIS** 38; © **Reuters/CORBIS** 173; © **Chico Sanchez/EFE/epa/CORBIS 6–7**; © **Kevin Schafer/CORBIS** 10–11, 16; © **Jim Sugar/CORBIS** 157b; © **Melvin G. Tarpley/US Army/ Handout/Reuters/CORBIS** 50a; © **Martin B. Withers/Frank Lane Picture Agency/CORBIS** 9a; **Hugh Cott,** *Adaptive Coloration in Animals,* **London 1940** 26, 29, 31, 32b, 33, 34; **Theodore Coulombe** 175;

Courtesy Arlene Elizabeth 178; **Mary Evans Picture Library** 36–37, 69a, 80, 81; **Courtesy Fat Ltd.** 188; **Courtesy F.O.A.** 189; **photograph © GLEN E. FRIEDMAN** – from the book *FUCK YOU HEROES* – **courtesy Burning Flags Press (www.BurningFlags.com)** 169; **Getty Images** 75a, 142a, 143; **Courtesy Graven Images Ltd.** 177b; **Fonds André Mare/IMEC** 72; **Courtesy Susan Keenes** 110l & r; **Kobal Collection** 162b; **Lehndorf and Trülzsch,** *Transfigurations,* **London 1986** 166; © **Claire Lieberman 2006, Photo Ken Kashian** 146–147, 182r; **Mark Lipson, courtesy Adelle Lutz** 8b; **Courtesy Lockheed Martin Corp.** 108a & b; **National Portrait Gallery, London** 88–89; © **the artists Courtesy Jay Jopling/White Cube (London)** 184r; **Courtesy Marilyn Lysohir** 179; **Maha Archive** 9r, 184l, 186; **Maha Archive, photo Laurie Bartley** 149; **Maha Archive, photo Neil Davenport** 174 ; **Maha Archive, photo Sam Handy** 177ar; **Photograph by Lee Miller © Lee Miller Archives, England 2006. All rights reserved. www.leemiller.co.uk** 92, 96l, 97, 117; **Photograph by David E. Scherman © Lee Miller Archives, England 2006. All rights reserved. www.leemiller.co.uk** 93; **Courtesy Aleksandra Mir** 185; **Courtesy NARA** 94r; **Tim Newark** 4–5, 40a, 43a, 45, 46a, 47, 56b, 65, 66–67, 137ar, 153l, 182l; **Courtesy James Cohan Gallery, New York** 180r; **The Metropolitan Museum of Art, New York, Gift of Michael Macko, 1991 (1991.35.1ab). Photograph 1995 The Metropolitan Museum of Art** 167; **Oxford Scientific Films** 35; © **Paris Musée de l'Armée, Dist. RMN © Pascal Segrette** 55al & ar, 56a, 82–83; **Edward Poulton,** *The Colours of Animals,* **London 1890** 14a, 23; **Courtesy RealTree** 51; **Courtesy Gerald Scarfe** 181b; **Courtesy Skate One Corporation** 177al & ac; **Courtesy Paul Smith** 170l & r; © **Margherita Spiluttini, courtesy Coop Himmelb(l)au** 187b; **Courtesy of the artist and Brändström & Stene Stockholm** 180l; **Courtesy Susumi Tachi** 162a; © **Tate, London 2002** 88a; **Courtesy Geoffrey (Tailor)'s Tartan Weaving Mill, Edinburgh** 40b; **Courtesy Sarah Taylor** 163r; **Abbott Thayer,** *Concealing Coloration in the Animal Kingdom,* **New York 1909** 19, 22, 24l; **U.S. Air Force photo** 157a, 160, 161b; **Courtesy U.S. Army** 156; © **Hundertwasser Archive, Vienna** 187a; **National Portrait Gallery, Smithsonian Institution, Washington, D.C.** 20; **Courtesy Yohji Yamamoto, photo Monica Feudi** 172r.

With thanks to Angela Godwin, Elizabeth Bowers, James Taylor, Gemma Maclagan, Peter Newark, Hardy Blechman, and the Collecting Departments of the Imperial War Museum.

Bibliography

Addison, G.H., *The Work of the Royal Engineers in the European War 1914–1918*, London, 1926

Lt-Col Armstrong, N.A.D., *Fieldcraft, Sniping and Intelligence*, Aldershot, 1940

'Art of Camouflage on Land and Sea', *The Sphere*, London, 3 August 1918, pp. 85–88

Beaver, M.D., and Borsarello, J.F., *Camouflage Uniforms of the Waffen SS*, Atglen, 1995

Behrens, R.R., *Art and Camouflage*, Cedar Falls, Iowa, 1981

Behrens, R.R., *False Colors: Art, Design and Modern Camouflage*, Dysart, Iowa, 2002

Bess, P., 'Infrared surveillance and Concealment', parts 1 and 2, *Military Illustrated*, issues 62 and 63, London, 1993

Blechman, H. (ed.), *DPM: An Encyclopaedia of Camouflage*, London, 2004

Borsarello, J.F., and Lassus, D., *Camouflaged Uniforms of the Waffen SS*, parts 1 and 2, London, 1988

Borsarello, J.F., *Camouflaged Uniforms of the NATO Forces*, London, 1989

Borsarello, J.F., *Camouflaged Uniforms of the Gulf and North African Forces*, London, 1989

Borsarello, J.F., and Kikuchi, A., *German Camouflage Uniforms 1937–1945*, Osaka, 1994

Brunel, G., 'Eugène Corbin, L'Inventeur du Camouflage en France', *Militaria Magazine*, Paris, September 2005

'Le Camouflage aux Armées', published in *La Guerre Documentée* by Lt-Col Le Marchand and Ernest Denis, Volume IV, Paris, c. 1920

Chesney, C.H.R., *The Art of Camouflage*, London, 1941

Chisolm, M., 'Experiment in Light and Shade', *Picture Post*, 17 November 1945

Cork, R., *A Bitter Truth: Avant-Garde Art and the Great War*, New Haven and London, 1994

Cott, H., *Adaptive Coloration in Animals*, London, 1940

Dobinson, C., *Fields of Deception: Britain's Bombing Decoys of World War II*, London, 2000

Friedmann, H., *The Natural-History Background of Camouflage*, Smithsonian Institution War Background Studies booklet No.5, Washington, December 1942

Greef, A.O., and Smith, A.J., *Evaluation of American Patterned Combat Uniforms*, Stores and Clothing Research and Development Establishment, Colchester, Essex, 1973

Hartcup, G., *Camouflage: A History of Concealment and Deception in War*, Newton Abbot, 1979

Hopkins, S., 'From "Cruel and Preposterous" to "Cool and Comfortably Clad"', *The Victorian Soldier*, National Army Museum, London, 1993

Latimer, J., *Deception in War*, London, 2001

Lehndorff, V., and Trülzsch, H., *Veruschka: Trans-figurations*, London, 1986

Maskelyne, J., *Magic: Top Secret*, London, 1949

Moran, J., 'US Marine Camouflage Uniforms 1942–45', parts 1,2 and 3, *Military Illustrated*, issues 32, 33 and 34, London, 1995

Musée de Bernay, *André Mare: Cubisme et Camouflage*, 1998

Newark, T., and Newark, Q., *Book of Camouflage*, London, 1996

Newark, T., *Book of Uniforms*, London, 1998

Newark, T., *The Future of Camouflage*, London, 2002

Penrose, A., *Roland Penrose: the Friendly Surrealist*, Munich and London, 2001

Penrose, R., *Home Guard Manual of Camouflage*, London, 1941

Penrose, R., *Picasso: His Life and Work*, London, 1958

Peterson, D., *Wehrmacht Camouflage Uniforms and Post-War Derivatives*, London, 1995

Peterson, D., *Waffen SS Camouflage Uniforms and Post-War Derivatives*, London, 1995

Poulton, E.G., *The Colours of Animals*, London, 1890

The Principles and Practice of Camouflage, issued by the General Staff, March 1918

Richardson, F.S., *Camouflage Fabrics both Plain and Printed for Military Use by the German SS and German Army*, 1945, reprinted London, 1988

Rudofsky, B., *Architecture Without Architects*, New York, 1965

Russell, L.E., 'Tigerstripe Camouflage of the Vietnam War', parts 1 and 2, *Military Illustrated*, issues 6 and 7, London, 1987

Solomon, S.J., *Strategic Camouflage*, London, 1920

Stanley II, R.M., *To Fool a Glass Eye: Camouflage versus Photoreconnaissance in World War II*, Shrewsbury, 1998

Stein, G., *The Autobiography of Alice B. Toklas*, London, 1933

Thayer, A.H., *Concealing Coloration in the Animal Kingdom*, London, 1909

Trevelyan, J., *Indigo Days*, London, 1957

Wilkinson, N., *The Dazzle Painting of Ships*, Newcastle-upon-Tyne, 1919

Wilkinson, N., *A Brush with Life*, London, 1969

VIZ, pamphlets on visual training for British military instructors, February–June issues, 1945

Windrow, M., 'Introduction to French Airborne Camouflage Uniforms, 1952–62', *Military Illustrated*, issue 16, London, 1989

Index